AF777865

Interferon 9

Interferon 9

1987

ION GRESSER
Editor-in-Chief

1987

ACADEMIC PRESS
Harcourt Brace Jovanovich, Publishers
London Orlando San Diego New York Austin
Boston Sydney Tokyo Toronto

ACADEMIC PRESS INC. (LONDON) LTD.
24/28 Oval Road
London NW1

United States Edition published by
ACADEMIC PRESS INC.
Orlando, Florida 32887

British Library Cataloguing in Publication Data

Interferon.——9 (1987)
1. Interferon——Periodicals
616.07′95 QR187.5

ISBN 0–12–302558–3

Typeset by Latimer Trend & Company Ltd, Plymouth
Printed in Great Britain at the Alden Press, Oxford

Contributors

A. Billiau, *Katholieke Universiteit Leuven, Rega Instituut, Mindrobroedersstraat 10, B-3000 Leuven, Belgium.*

G. Buchan, *The Charing Cross Sunley Research Centre, Lurgan Avenue, Hammersmith, London W6 8LW*

M. Feldman, *The Charing Cross Sunley Research Centre, Lurgan Avenue, Hammersmith, London W6 8LW*

M. Hirsch, *Infectious Disease Unit, Massachusetts General Hospital, Fruit Street, Boston, MA 02114, USA.*

S. L. Lin, *The Rockefeller University, 1230 York Avenue, New York, NY 10021, USA*

M. Londei, *The Charing Cross Sunley Research Centre, Lurgan Avenue, Hammersmith, London W8 8LW*

L. M. Pfeffer, *The Rockefeller University, 1230 York Avenue, New York, NY 10021, USA*

R. J. Pomerantz, *Infectious Disease Unit, Massachusetts General Hospital, Fruit Street, Boston, MA 02114, USA.*

P. B. Sehgal, *The Rockefeller University, 1230 York Avenue, New York, NY 10021, USA*

I. Tamm, *The Rockefeller University, 1230 York Avenue, New York, NY 10021, USA*

K. C. Zoon, *Division of Virology, Office of Biologics Research & Review, Centre for Drugs and Biologics, 8800 Rockville Pike, Building 29A, Bethesda, MD 20205, USA.*

Contents

Interferons and Autoimmunity

Marc Feldmann, Marco Londei and Glenn Buchan

The Interferon–Interleukin 1 Connection

A. Billiau

Interferon and Human Immunodeficiency Virus Infection

Roger J. Pomerantz and Martin S. Hirsch

Human Interferons: Structure and Function

KATHRYN C. ZOON

Division of Virology, Office of Biologics Research and Review, Center for Drugs and Biologics, Food and Drug Administration, 8800 Rockville Pike, Bethesda, MD 20892

I INTRODUCTION

The structure and function of interferon (IFN) has been a subject of interest since its discovery in 1957 (Isaacs and Lindenmann, 1957). However, it was not until the second half of the 1970s, with the successful purification of several natural IFNs, that we could start asking questions on the relationship between the structure of IFN and its resulting biological activities (review, Lengyel, 1982). The recent revolution in recombinant DNA technology and its application to the production of large quantities of many of the naturally occurring IFN species, as well as of unique hybrid forms of these molecules, has greatly contributed to our knowledge of the chemistry and biology of IFNs. Today, we have a great deal of structural information on these molecules at our disposal from a variety of chemical and physical techniques.

INTERFERON 9
ISBN 0 12 302558 3

This article summarizes our present state of knowledge of human IFN structure and its relationship to molecular action.

II NOMENCLATURE AND CHEMICAL PROPERTIES OF HUMAN IFNs

IFNs were originally classified based on the cell types from which they were derived, their chemical properties, and their antigenicity (Stewart *et al.*, 1980). With the cloning of a number of IFN molecules and our increasing knowledge of IFN structure, the nomenclature of IFN has also evolved. Today, three major classes of IFN have been designated, IFN-α, IFN-β, and IFN-γ (Table 1). Human IFN-α and -β_1 are approximately 30% similar at the primary amino acid sequence level, while IFN-γ is similar to neither (reviews, Zoon and Wetzel, 1984; Langer and Pestka, 1985).

Human IFN-α is actually a family of IFN species. More than 24 species have been identified so far, from gene and protein sequence data (Pestka, 1986; Weissmann and Weber, 1986; Zoon and Wetzel, 1984). Only one major species of human IFN-β (IFN-β_1) has been isolated (Taniguchi *et al.*, 1979; Knight *et al.*, 1980); however, recently a second form of IFN derived from human fibroblasts has been described and is at present designated IFN-β_2 (Revel *et al.*, 1986; Haegeman *et al.*, 1986). Only a single gene has been found for human IFN-γ, although multiple protein species have been identified (Gray *et al.*, 1982; Rinderknecht *et al.*, 1984). These species are the result of post-translational modification (Rinderknecht *et al.*, 1984). The genes for human IFN-α and -β_1 are located on chromosome 9 (Owerbach *et al.*, 1981), while the gene for human IFN-γ is found on chromosome 12 (Naylor *et al.*, 1983). Naturally occurring human IFN-β and -γ are glycosylated proteins (Knight and Fahey, 1982; Rinderknecht *et al.*, 1984). Human IFN-α species were generally considered not to be glycosylated (review, Lengyel, 1982); however, recent evidence suggests that several species are glycosylated (Labdon *et al.*, 1984; Zoon *et al.*, in press). In

TABLE I Nomenclature and Properties of Human Interferons

Class	Alpha	Beta	Gamma
Number of species	$\geqslant 24$	2	1
Glycosylation	$\geqslant 3$ species	yes	yes
Apparent MW	16,000–27,000	20,000	15,500–25,000
Disulphide bonds	2	1	0
Number of amino acids	165–166	166	143
Chromosome coding for IFN	9	9	12

general, human IFN-α species and human IFN-β are stable to pH 2 treatment, while human IFN-γ is not. However, it should be pointed out that one recent report states that up to 40% of the human IFN-α derived from peripheral blood lymphocytes is acid labile (Chada, 1985).

III STRUCTURE AND FUNCTION

A Human IFN-α

Human IFN-α was believed to be a heterogenous population of molecules even before its purification to homogeneity, because of its physicochemical properties as studied by isoelectric focusing, sodium dodecyl sulphate polyacrylamide gel electrophoresis (SDS PAGE) and affinity chromatography (reviews, Lengyel, 1982; Langer and Pestka, 1985). In the late 1970s, when IFN-α was finally purified using a variety of techniques, including high performance liquid chromatography (HPLC) (Rubinstein *et al.*, 1979) and SDS PAGE (Zoon *et al.*, 1979), this hypothesis was confirmed. So far, multiple species of human IFN-α have been purified and partially characterized from virus-induced chronic myelogenous leukaemia (CML) cells (10 species) (Rubinstein *et al.*, 1981), KG-1 cells (9 species) (Hobbs and Pestka, 1982), Namalwa cells (18 species) (Zoon *et al.*, 1985, 1986, in press; Allen, 1982), and normal peripheral blood lymphocytes (23 species) (K. Zoon, unpublished results). The apparent molecular weights range from 16,000 to 27,000 (Zoon *et al.*, 1979, 1980, 1982, 1985, 1986; Allen, 1982; Rubinstein *et al.*, 1981; Hobbs and Pestka, 1982). The amino acid compositions of these natural IFNs are very similar; the amino acid sequences of these IFN-α species are also similar (> 50%) among themselves but do exhibit sequence differences (Zoon *et al.*, 1979, 1980, 1982, 1985, 1986; Allen, 1982; Rubinstein *et al.*, 1981; Hobbs and Pestka, 1982; reviews, Zoon and Wetzel, 1984; Langer and Pestka, 1985).

Since the application of recombinant DNA technology to the cloning of IFN genes, the primary amino acid sequences of at least 24 species have been deduced from the gene sequences (Fig. 1). Those genes which are closely related are indicated in parentheses; small differences do exist between several of these essentially identical species, e.g., IFN-αA* has a lysine at position 23 while IFN-α_2 has an arginine at this position. Other differences between similar species have been summarized in recent reviews (Pestka, 1986; Weissmann and Weber, 1986). The molecular weights of the recombinant human IFN-α species range from 19,241 to 19,745, based on their

*IFN-αA is now designated IFN-α_{2a} and IFN-α_2 is now designated IFN-α_{2b}.

AMINO ACID SEQUENCES OF HUMAN IFN-α SPECIES

	S1–S10	S20	S23	1–10	20	30	40	50	60	70
IFN-α consensus	MALSFSLLMA	VLVLSYKSIC	SLG	CDLPQTHSLG	NRRALILLAQ	MGRISPFSCL	KDRHDFGFPQ	EEFDGNQFQK	AQAISVLHEM	IQQTFNLFST
IFN-αK (α6)	...P.A....	LV...C..S.	..D	....	H..TMM....	.R...L....	......R...	....	.E.......V	....
IFN-α5 (αG)	...P.V....	LV..NC....	...	.........S	...T.MIM..	....	....	....	....	....
IFN-αA (α2)	...T.A..V.	L....C..S.	.V.	....	S..T.M....	.RK..L....	....	...-......	.ET.P.....	...I......
IFN-αD (α1)	..SP.A...V	LV...C..S.	...	....E....D	...T.M....	.S....S...	M.........	....	.P.......L	...I....T.
IFN-αH1 (αH2)	...P...M..	LV...C..S.	...	.N.S.....N	...T.M.M..	.R........	......E...	....	....	M.........
IFN-αB2 (α8)	...T.Y..V.	LV......FS	...	....	....	.R........	......E...	....DK....	....	....
IFN-αB	...T.Y.MV.	LV......FS	...	....	....	.R........	......E...	....DK....	....	....
IFN-α4b	....	....	...	....	....	.....H....	.........E	.....H....	T.........	....
IFN-αC	....	....	...	....	........G.	....	......RI..	....	....	....
IFN-αL (Ψα10)	....	.........*	...	........T.R	........G.	....	......RI..	....	....	....
IFN-αJ1 (α7)	..R......V	....	...	.........R	....	....	....E.R..E	.....H....	T.........	....
IFN-αJ2	..R......V	....	...	.........R	....	....	....E.R..E	.....H....	T.........	....
IFN-αI	....	....	...	....	....	....	...P...L..	....	T.........	....
IFN-αF	....	....	...	....	....	....	....	....	....	....
IFN-αWA	....	....	...	....	....	.....H....	...Y......	.V........	.....AF...	....
IFN-αGx-1	...P...M..	LV...C..S.	...	.N.S.....N	...T.MIM..	....	....	....	....	....
IFN-α76	....	....	...	....	....	.....H....	.........E	.....H....	....	....
IFN-α88		....	...	....	....	....	.......L..	....	T.........	....

	80	90	100	110	120	130	140	150	160	166
IFN-α consensus	KDSSAAWDES	LLEKFSTELY	QQLNDLEACV	IQEVGVEETP	LMNEDSILAV	RKYFQRITLY	LTEKKYSPCA	WEVVRAEIMR	SFSFSTNLQK	RLRRKD
IFN-αK (α6)	....V....R	..D.LY....	....	M...W.GG..	....	....	....	....	...S.R...E	.....E
IFN-αG (α5)	.....T...T	..D..Y....	.........M	M......D..	...V....T.	....	....	....	...L.A...E	.....E
IFN-αA (α2)	.........T	..D..Y....	....	..G...T...	..K.......	....	.K........	....	...L.....E	S..S.E
IFN-αD (α1)	.........D	..D..C....	....	M..ER.G...	...V......	K...R.....	....	....	.L.L.....E	.....E
IFN-αH1 (αH2)	.N.......T	.....YI..F	..M.......	....	....	K.........	.M........	....	....	......
IFN-αB2 (α8)	......L..T	..DE.YI..D	.......S..	M.....I.S.	..Y.......	....	.......S..	....	...L.I....	..KS.E
IFN-αB	......L..T	..DE.YI..D	VLC	D.....I.S.	..Y.......	....	.......S..	....	...L.I....	..KS.E
IFN-α4b	E......EQ.	....	....	....	...V......	....	....	....	.L........	......
IFN-αC	E......EQ.	....	....	....	....	....	.I.R......	....	.L........	......
IFN-αL (Ψα10)	E......EQ.	........I.	....	....	....	....	.I.R......	....	.L........	......
IFN-αJ1 (α7)	E......EQ.	....	....	....	.....F....	....	.M........	....	........K.	G.....
IFN-αJ2	E......EQ.	....	....	....	.....F....	....	.M........	....	....	......
IFN-αI	E......EQ.	....	....N.....	.....M....	....	....	....	....	.L........	I.....
IFN-αF	.....T.EQ.	.........N	.....M....	....	...V......	K.........	....	....	...L.KIF.E	.....E
IFN-αWA	.........T	..D..YI..F	....	T.......IA	....	....	.MG.......	....	....	G.....
IFN-αGx-1	.....T...T	..D..Y....	.........M	M......D..	...V....T.	....	....	....	...L.A...E	.....E
IFN-α76	E......EQ.	....	....	....	....	....	....	....	.L........	......
IFN-α88	E......EQ	....	....N.....	.....M....	....	....	....	....	.L........	......

amino acid compositions (Langer and Pestka, 1985). Most of these species have a signal peptide sequence of 23 amino acid residues and a mature amino acid sequence of 166 amino acid residues, although human IFN-α_2 has 165 residues and human IFN-α_{II}1 (not shown), 172 residues. Approximately 50% (85/166) of the residues of the mature sequence are identical and many of the substitutions are conservative.

The region between 139 to 151 is strongly conserved among the IFN-α species and IFN-β (see Figs 1 and 2). Most of the IFN-α species have four conserved cysteines at positions 1, 29, 98/99 and 138/139. Human IFN-α_1, which is essentially the same as IFN-α_{13} and IFN-αD, has an additional cysteine at position 86. Disulphide bonds were shown to be formed between residues 1 and 98/99, and 29 and 138/139, in IFN-αA (Wetzel, 1981). Studies using chemical derivatization (Morehead *et al.*, 1984) and site specific mutagenesis (De Chiara *et al.*, 1986) indicated that the 1 to 98/99 disulphide bond is not essential for maintaining the biologically active conformation of IFN-α_2.

Some of the natural human IFN-α species appear to have sequences as determined by amino acid sequence analysis that are different from those deduced from the cDNA or gene sequences. One species, derived from virus-induced Namalwa cells, has an asparagine at position 5 which has not been observed in the sequences of recombinant DNA-derived IFNs (K. Zoon, unpublished results). In addition, two of the fully active IFN-α species isolated from CML cells consist of only 155 amino acids; they lack the last 10 *C*-terminal amino acid residues (Levy *et al.*, 1981). This study also showed that these 10 residues are not essential for biological activity. Similarly, recombinant DNA-derived human IFN-α_2 lacking the *C*-terminal 13 amino acid residues, prepared by limited proteolysis, was also fully active (Wetzel *et al.*, 1982; Chang *et al.*, 1982). Furthermore, an antibody which binds to residues 151–166 of human IFN-α_2 can recognize IFN-α_2 bound to its receptor (Arnheiter *et al.*, 1983). These data indicate that the *C* terminus is not involved in binding of the IFN to its receptor and is not necessary for eliciting maximum biological activity. Although there is some confusion as to which amino acid is at position 1 for the naturally derived human IFN-α species, the first residue is probably a cysteine as determined by reduction and alkylation studies (Allen and Fantes, 1980).

Fig. 1 Protein sequences of HuIFN-alphas deduced from cDNA or genomic DNA sequences. S1 etc. indicate signal peptide amino acid residues. Corresponding residues are presented only when they differ from the consensus sequence. Residues which are common to all listed sequences are underlined in the consensus sequence. Sequences A-L are from the laboratories of Pestka, Goeddel, and colleagues, whereas sequences with numeric designations are from the laboratory of Weissman and colleagues (Goeddel *et al.*, 1980; Goeddel *et al.*, 1981; Lawn *et al.*, 1981; Mantei *et al.*, 1980; Streuli *et al.*, 1980; Weissmann and Weber, 1986). From Pestka (1986); reprinted with permission from the author.

The predicted secondary structure of several IFN-α species is shown in Fig. 2. These molecules were calculated to have a large α-helix content and essentially no β-sheet. This estimate was confirmed by circular dichroism studies of human IFN-α_2, in which the α-helix content was estimated to be 45–70% and the β-sheet content 0% (Bewley *et al.*, 1982). Structural studies of human IFN-α_2, employing Raman spectroscopy, indicated 49% α-helix, 25% disordered helix, 8% extended β-sheet and 10% turns (Zoon and Wetzel, 1984). Target analysis of human IFN-α suggests that the functional unit is a monomer (Rehberg *et al.*, 1982). Although crystals of human IFN-α_2 have been obtained (Nagabhushan *et al.*, 1984; Miller *et al.*, 1982), tertiary structure results are still pending.

In the past, the presence of carbohydrate on human IFN-α species has been a controversial issue (Lengyel, 1982). However, recently it was demonstrated that several species from CML, KG-1 and Namalwa (Labdon *et al.*, 1984; Zoon *et al.*, in press) cells are indeed glycosylated. The natures of the structure and linkage of the carbohydrate to the IFN-α species are unknown: however, it is postulated that the sugar moiety is covalently linked to the protein by 0-glycosylation, because all but one of the human IFN-α sequences lack the Asn-X-Ser/Thr sequence which is necessary for *N*-glycosylation.

B Human IFN-β

Natural human IFN-β (IFN-β_1), a glycoprotein, was first purified to homogeneity in 1976 from human diploid fibroblasts (Knight, 1976). Subsequently, a number of purification schemes have been devised and limited *N*-terminal amino acid sequence data have become available (up to 19 residues) (Knight *et al.*, 1980; Okamura *et al.*, 1980; Stein *et al.*, 1980; Freisen *et al.*, 1981). Recently, a second human β-like IFN (IFN-β_2) was reported which differs from human IFN-β_1 in its sequence, biochemical and immunochemical properties, although one neutralizing monoclonal which binds to IFN-β_1 also neutralizes the antiviral activity of IFN-β_2 (Zilberstein *et al.*, 1986; Revel *et al.*, 1986; Haegeman *et al.*, 1986). This second IFN-β-like molecule represents approximately 5% of the IFN secreted by poly(I:C)-superinduced diploid fibroblasts.

The complete amino acid sequence of human IFN-β_1 as derived from the cDNA sequence is shown in Fig. 3 (Taniguchi *et al.*, 1979). It has a molecular weight of 20,027 and is made up of a mature protein of 166 amino acid residues and a signal peptide of 21 amino acids. Human IFN-β_1 has three cysteines at positions 17, 31 and 141. The limited amino acid sequence data for natural human IFN-β_1 is in complete agreement with the amino acid sequence deduced from the cDNA sequence. The recombinant DNA analo-

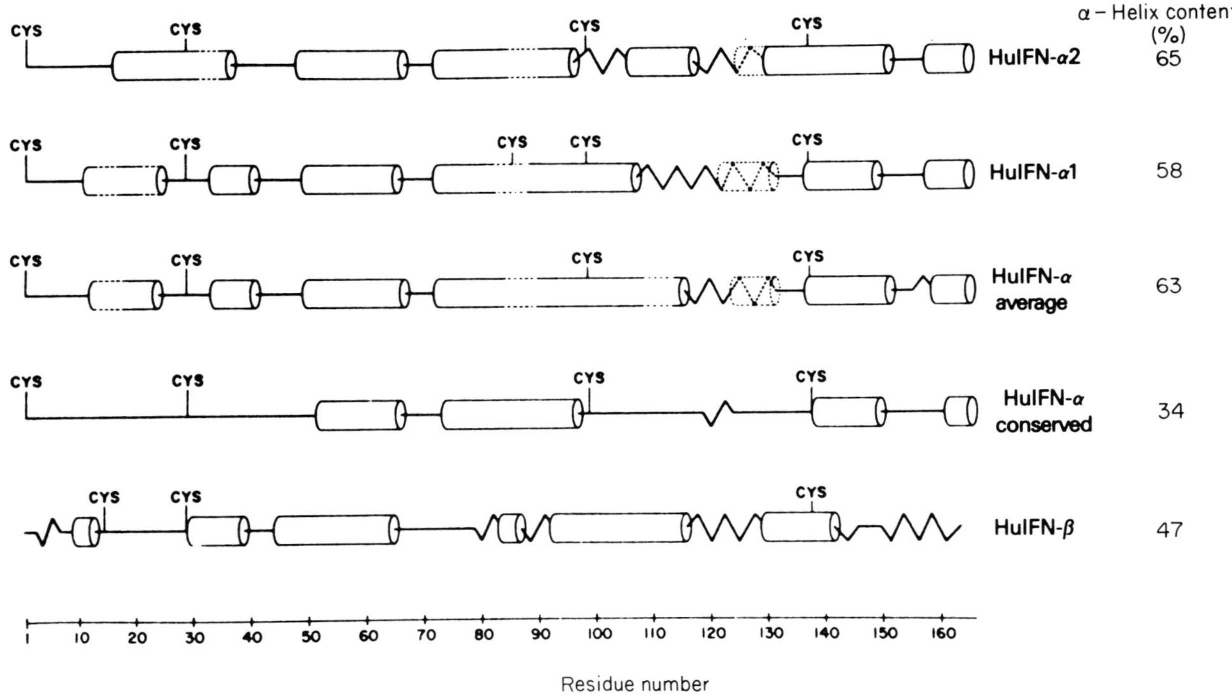

Fig. 2 Secondary structure predictions for HuIFN-α and HuIFN-β applying the algorithm of Garnier *et al.* (1978) to amino acid sequences predicted from sequences of cloned cDNA. Residues were scored for their relative tendencies to exist in four possible states (α-helix, extended chain, reverse turn, and coil) based on values for each amino acid obtained by examination of 26 protein crystal structures. Only α-helix (barrels) and extended chain (β-sheet, zigzags) are shown since they are predicted most accurately. Stretches equally likely to be in α-helix or extended chain are shown with these structures dotted and superimposed. Regions with moderate helical potential which might be strengthened by adjoining helical regions are shown as dotted connections between helices. From Zoon and Wetzel (1984); reprinted with permission from Springer-Verlag.

```
S1               S10                 S20  1                 10                  20                  30                 40
M T N K C L L Q I A L L L C F S T T A L S M S Y N L L G F L Q R S S N F Q C Q K L L W Q L N G R L E Y C L K D R M N F D I

                 50                  60                  70                  80                  90                 100
P E E I K Q L Q Q F Q K E D A A L T I Y E M L Q N I F A I F R Q D S S S T G W N E T I V E N L L A N V Y H Q I N H L K T V L E

               110                 120                 130                 140                 150                 160
E K L E K E D F T R G K L M S S L H L K R Y Y G R I L H Y L K A K E Y S H C A W T I V R V E I L R N F Y F I N R L T G Y L R N
```

Fig. 3 Protein sequence of HuIFN-β deduced from nucleotide sequence. S1 etc. indicate signal peptide amino acid residues. From Zoon and Wetzel (1984); reprinted with permission from Springer-Verlag.

gue of IFN-β_1, [Ser^{17}]IFN-β, which exhibits essentially the same specific activity as that of natural IFN-β_1 (1.1×10^8 U/mg protein), suggests that the cysteine at position 17 is not involved in a disulphide linkage and this cysteine is not essential for its biological properties (Khosrovi, 1984). However, in contrast, another analogue, [Tyr^{141}]IFN-β, has essentially no antiviral activity (Shepard *et al.*, 1981). Thus, this evidence suggests that the Cys 31 and Cys 141 form a disulphide bond which is essential for its biological activity. The predicted secondary structure for human IFN-β is shown in Fig. 2. The α-helix content appears to be less than that of the IFN-α species (47%). Circular dichroism studies of human IFN-β_1 indicate that it has an α-helix content of 55% (M. Boublik and H. Kung, personal communication). Target analysis of HuIFN-β suggests that the functional unit is a dimer (Rehberg *et al.*, 1982).

IFN-β_1 has been clearly demonstrated to be a glycoprotein (Knight and Fahey, 1982). The carbohydrate is believed to be linked to the Asn at position 80 by *N*-glycosylation. Treatment of natural IFN-β with a mixture of glycosidases resulted in a shift in the apparent molecular weight from 23,000 to 18,000. At present, no information is available on the tertiary structure of this molecule.

C Human IFN-γ

The purification of human IFN-γ derived from peripheral blood lymphocytes was originally reported in 1982 (Yip *et al.*, 1982) and more recently in 1984 (Rinderknecht *et al.*, 1984). The complete primary amino acid sequence of two forms (25 KD and 20 KD) of naturally occurring IFN-γ revealed that there was one primary amino acid sequence (Fig. 4). However, two sites of *N*-glycosylation were observed in the sequence, and the two forms were found to differ in their degrees of glycosylation. The 25 KD species appears to be glycosylated at both Asn 25 and Asn 97 while the 20 KD species is glycosylated only at Asn 97. Both forms exhibited a great deal of heterogeneity at the *C*-terminus, i.e., truncated *C*-termini at positions 127, 128, 129, 130, 132 and 134 (see Fig. 4) (Rinderknecht *et al.*, 1984). Recombinant DNA-derived IFN-γ lacking the residues Cys-Tyr-Cys at the *N*-terminus has a molecular weight of 16,757. The amino acid sequence of human IFN-γ deduced from the cDNA was in agreement with that of natural human IFN-γ (Fig. 4). Some minor heterogeneity has been reported in the cDNA sequence which codes for the amino acid residue at position 140; in one case the cDNA codes for a glutamine (Gray *et al.*, 1982) and in the other it codes for an arginine (Gray and Goeddel, 1982; Devos *et al.*, 1982). Recombinant human IFN-γ also undergoes processing of its *C*-terminus when expressed in *E. coli*. Removal of four amino acids from the *C*-terminus does not affect the antiviral or antiproliferative activities; however, deletion of 19 *C*-terminal amino acids by recombinant DNA technology resulted in a 1000-fold decrease in antiviral and antiproliferative specific activities (Czarniecki *et al.*, 1985). From the original recombinant DNA studies, it was reported that IFN-γ was made up of a signal peptide of 20 amino acid residues and a mature protein of 146 amino acid residues. The assignment of Cys-Tyr-Cys as residues 1–3 was based to some extent on analogy with the cysteine at position 1 of the human IFN-α species. One discrepancy which was cleared up as a result of obtaining the amino acid sequence of natural IFN-γ was that the first residue of the *N*-terminus of IFN-γ was glutamic acid in the form of pyroglutamate (see Fig. 4). Supporting evidence for this assignment was the observation that recombinant DNA-derived IFN-γ obtained from COS-7

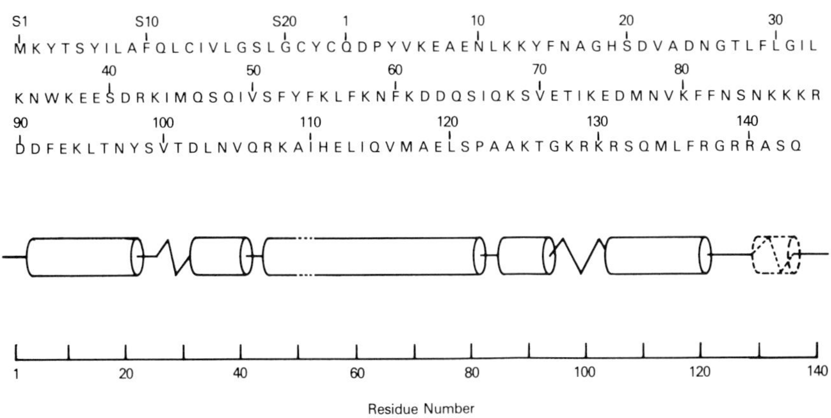

Fig. 4 The protein sequence of HuIFN-γ deduced from the nucleotide sequence, and the secondary structure prediction for HuIFN-γ using the algorithm of Garnier *et al.*, 1978. (See Fig. 2.) From Zoon and Wetzel (1984); reprinted with permission from Springer-Verlag.

cells lacked the Cys-Try-Cys residues and had a blocked *N*-terminus, pyroglutamate (Rinderknecht *et al.*, 1984). Thus, it appears that the mature human IFN-γ protein has no cysteine residues, and it follows that disulphide bonds do not exist in this molecule. It should also be noted that human IFN-γ contains an acid-labile Asp-Pro bond between positions 2 and 3. Treatment at pH 2.3 for 30 minutes at 100°C breaks the Asp-Pro bond and the IFN-γ loses 100% of its antiviral activity (M. Rubinstein, personal communication). Target analysis of human IFN-γ suggested that the functional unit is a tetramer (Rehberg *et al.*, 1982); however, gel filtration studies suggest the natural state of IFN-γ to be a dimer (Rinderknecht *et al.*, 1984). Again, as with the other human IFNs, the tertiary structure of IFN-γ is as yet unknown.

IV SUMMARY

Other relevant areas of research regarding the structure and function of IFNs include the study of IFN fragments and hybrid IFN molecules prepared by recombinant DNA technology, and monoclonal antibodies against IFNs have also made major contributions to our knowledge of IFN structure and function. However, these topics have been addressed in a number of recent reviews (Zoon and Wetzel, 1984; Langer and Pestka, 1985). We are now awaiting the crystal structure of several human IFNs. Once this knowledge has been acquired, we can proceed to envisage at the three-dimensional level how these molecules interact with their receptors to produce their numerous biological activities.

REFERENCES

Allen, G. (1982). *Biochem. J.* **207**, 397–408.

Allen, G. and Fantes, K. H. (1980). *Nature (London)* **287**, 408–411.

Arnheiter, H., Ohno, M., Smith, M., Gutte, B. and Zoon, K. C. (1983). *Proc. Natl Acad. Sci. USA* **80**, 2539–2543.

Berg, K. and Heron, I. (1980). *Scand. J. Immunol.* **11**, 489–502.

Bewley, T. A., Levine, H. L. and Wetzel, R. (1982). *Int. J. Peptide Protein Res.* **20**, 93–96.

Chada, K. C. (1985). *In* "The Interferon System" (F. Dianzani and G. B. Rossi, eds), pp. 35–41. Raven Press, New York.

Chang, N. T., Kung, H.-F. and Pestka, S. (1982). *Arch. Biochem. Biophys.* **221**, 585–589.

Czarniecki, C. W., Burton, L. E. and Rinderknecht, E. (1985). *In* The 1985 TNO-ISIR Meeting on the Interferon System, Clearwater Beach, Florida, USA, 13–18 October.

De Chiara, T. M., Erlitz, F. and Tarnowski, S. J. (1986). *Meth. Enzym.* **119**, 403–415.

Devos, R., Cheroutre, H., Taya, Y., Degrave, W., Van Heuverswyn, H. and Fiers, W. (1982). *Nucleic Acids Res.* **10**, 2487–2501.

Friesen, H.-J., Stein, S., Evinger, M., Familletti, P. C., Moschera, J., Meienhofer, J., Shively, J. and Pestka, S. (1981). *Arch. Biochem. Biophys.* **206**, 432–450.

Garnier, J., Osguthorpe, D. J. and Robson, B. (1978). *J. Mol. Biol.* **120**, 97–120.

Gray, P. W. and Goeddel, D. V. (1982). *Nature* **298**, 859–863.

Gray, P. W., Leung, D. W., Pennica, D., Yelverton, E., Najarian, R., Simonsen, C. C., Derynck, R., Sherwood, P. J., Wallace, D. M., Berger, S. L., Levinson, A. D. and Goeddel, D. V. (1982). *Nature* **295**, 503–508.

Goeddel, D. V., Yelverton, E., Ullrich, A., Heyneker, H. L., Miozzari, G., Holmes, W., Seeburg, P. H., Dull, T., May, L., Stebbing, N., Crea, R., Maeda, S., McCandliss, R., Sloma, A., Tabor, J. M., Gross, M., Familletti, P. C. and Pestka, S. (1980). *Nature (London)* **287**, 411–416.

Goeddel, D. V., Leung, D. W., Dull, T. J., Gross, M., Lawn, R. M., McCandliss, R., Seeburg, P. H., Ullrich, A., Yelverton, E. and Gray, P. W. (1981). *Nature (London)* **290**, 20–26.

Haegeman, G., Content, J., Volckaert, G., Derynck, R., Tavernier, J., Fiers, W. (1986). *Eur. J. Biochem.* **159,** 625–632.

Hobbs, D. S. and Pestka, S. (1982). *J. Biol. Chem.* **257**, 4071–4076.

Isaacs, A. and Lindenmann, J. (1957). *Proc. R. Soc. Lond., Ser. B* **147,** 258–267.

Khosrovi, B. (1984). *In* "Interferon: Research, Clinical Application, and Regulatory Consideration" (K. C. Zoon, P. Noguchi and T.-Y. Liu, eds), pp. 89–99. Elsevier Science Publishing Co., Amsterdam.

Knight, E., Jr (1976). *Proc. Natl Acad. Sci. USA* **73**, 520–523.

Knight, E., Jr and Fahey, D. (1982). *J. Interferon Res.* **2**, 421–429.

Knight, E., Jr, Hunkapiller, M. W., Korant, B. D., Hardy, R. W. F. and Hood, L. E. (1980). *Science* **207**, 525–526.

Labdon, J. E., Gibson, K. D., Sun, S. and Pestka, S. (1984). *Arch. Biochem. Biophys.* **232**, 422–426.

Langer, J. A. and Pestka, S. (1985). *Pharmac. Ther.* **27**, 371–401.

Lawn, R. M., Adelman, J., Dull, T. J., Gross, M., Goeddel, D. V. and Ullrich, A. (1981a). *Science* **212**, 1159–1162.

Lengyel, P. (1982). *Ann. Rev. Biochem.* **51**, 251–282.

Levy, W. P., Rubinstein, M., Shively, J., Del Valle, U., Lai, C.-Y., Moschera, J., Brink, L., Gerber, L., Stein, S. and Pestka, S. (1981). *Proc. Natl Acad. Sci. USA* **78**, 6186–6190.

Mantei, N., Schwarzstein, M., Streuli, M., Panem, S., Nagata, S. and Weissmann, C. (1980). *Gene* **10**, 1–10.

Miller, D. L., Kung, H.-F. and Pestka, S. (1982). *Science* **215**, 689–690.

Morehead, H., Johnston, P. D. and Wetzel, R. (1984). *Biochemistry* **23**, 2500–2507.

Nagabhushan, T. L., Surprenant, H., Le, H. V., Kosecki, R., Levine, A., Reichert, P., Sharma, B., Tsai, H., Trotta, P., Bausch, J., Foster, C., Gruber, S., Hoogerheide, J. and Mercorelli, S. (1984). *In* "Interferon: Research, Clinical Application, and Regulatory Consideration" (K. Zoon, P. Noguchi and T.-Y. Liu, eds), pp. 79–88. Elsevier Science Publishing Co., Amsterdam.

Naylor, S. L., Sakaguchi, A. Y., Shows, T. B., Law, M. L., Goeddel, D. V. and Gray, P. W. (1983). *J. Exp. Med.* **157**, 1020–1027.

Okamura, H., Berthold, W., Hood, L., Hunkapiller, M., Inoue, M., Smith-Johannsen, H. and Tan, Y. H. (1980). *Biochemistry* **19**, 3831–3835.

Owerbach, D., Rutter, W. J., Shows, T. B., Gray, P., Goeddel, D. V. and Lawn, R. M. (1981). *Proc. Natl Acad. Sci. USA* **78**, 3123–3127.

Pestka, S. (1986). *Meth. Enzym.* **119**, 3–14.

Rehberg, E., Kelder, B., Hoal, E. G. and Pestka, S. (1982). *J. Biol. Chem.* **257**, 11497–11502.

Revel, M., Ruggieri, R. and Zilberstein, A. (1986). *In* "The Biology of the Interferon System 1985" (W. E. Stewart II and H. Schellekesn, eds), pp. 207–216. Elsevier Science Publishers B.V., Amsterdam.

Rinderknecht, E., O'Connor, B. H. and Rodriquez, H. (1984). *J. Biol. Chem.* **259**, 6790–6797.

Rubinstein, M., Levy, W. P., Moschera, J. A., Lai, C.-Y., Hershberg, R. D., Bartlett, R. T. and Pestka, S. (1981). *Arch. Biochem. Biophys.* **210**, 307–318.

Rubinstein, M., Rubinstein, S., Familletti, P. C., Miller, R. S., Waldman, A. A. and Pestka, S. (1979). *Proc. Natl Acad. Sci. USA* **76**, 640–644.

Shepard, H. M., Leung, D. W., Stebbing, N. and Goeddel, D. V. (1981). *Nature* **294**, 563–565.

Stein, S., Kenny, C., Friesen, H.-J., Shively, J., Del Valle, U. and Pestka, S. (1980). *Proc. Natl Acad. Sci. USA* **77**, 5716–5719.

Stewart II, W. E., Blalock, J. E., Burke, D. C., Chany, C., Dunnick, J., Falcoff, E., Friedman, R. M., Galasso, G. J., Joklik, W. K., Vilcek, J. T., Younger, J. S. and Zoon, K. C. (1980). *Nature* **286**, 110.

Streuli, M., Nagata, S. and Weissmann, C. (1980). *Science* **209**, 1343–1347.

Taniguchi, T., Sakai, M., Fujii-Kuriyama, Y., Muramatsu, M., Kobayashi, S. and Sudo, T. (1979). *Proc. Jap. Acad.* **B55**, 464–469.

Weissmann, C. and Weber, H. (1986). *Prog. Nuc. Acid Res. Molec. Biol.* **33**, 251–300.

Wetzel, R. (1981). *Nature* **289**, 606–607.

Wetzel, R., Levine, H. L., Estell, D. A., Shire, S., Finer-Moore, J., Stroud, R. M. and Bewley, T. A. (1982). *In* "Chemistry and Biology of Interferons: Relationship to Therapeutics" (T. Merigan, R. Friedman and C. F. Fox, eds), pp. 365–376. Academic Press, New York.

Yip, Y. K., Barrowclough, B. S., Urban, C. and Vilcek, J. (1982). *Proc. Natl Acad. Sci. USA* **79**, 1820–1824.

Zilberstein, A., Nissim, A., Ruggieri, R., Shulman, L., Chen, L. and Revel, M. (1986). *In* "The Biology of the Interferon System 1985" (W. E. Stewart II and H. Schellekens, eds), pp. 119–124. Elsevier Science Publishers B. V., Amsterdam.

Zoon, K. C. and Wezel, R. (1984). *In* "Handbook of Exp. Pharmacol. 71" (P. E. Came and W. A. Carter, eds), pp. 79–100. Springer-Verlag, Berlin.

Zoon, K. C., Smith, M. E., Bridgen, P. J., Zur Nedden, D. and Anfinsen, C. B. (1979). *Proc. Natl Acad. Sci. USA* **76**, 5601–5605.

Zoon, K. C., Smith, M. E., Bridgen, P. J. and Anfinsen, C. B. (1980). *Science* **207**, 527–528.

Zoon, K. C., Miller, D., Zur Nedden, D. and Hunkapiller, M. W. (1982). *J. Interferon Res.* **2**, 253–260.

Zoon, K. C., Hu, R.-Q., Zur Nedden, D. and Nguyen, N. (1985). *In* "The Biology of the Interferon System 1984" (H. Kirchner and H. Schellekens, eds), pp. 61–67. Elsevier, Amsterdam.

Zoon, K. C., Hu, R.-Q., Zur Nedden, D., Gerrard, T. L., Enterline, J. E., Boykins, R. A. and Nguyen, N. Y. (1986). *In* "The Biology of the Interferon System 1985" (E. W. Stewart II and H. Schellekens, eds), pp. 55–58. Elsevier Science Publishers B. V., Amsterdam.

Zoon, K. C., Zur Nedden, D. L., Enterline, J. C., Manischewitz, J., Dyer, D. R., Boykins, R. A., Bekisz, J. and Gerrard, T. L. (1987). *In* "The Biology of the Interferon System 1986" (K. Cantell and H. Schellekens, eds). Martinus Nijhoff Publishers, Amsterdam. In press.

Interferons α and β as Cellular Regulatory Molecules

IGOR TAMM, STANLEY L. LIN, LAWRENCE M. PFEFFER, PRAVINKUMAR B. SEHGAL

The Rockefeller University, 1230 York Avenue, New York, NY 10021, USA

INTERFERON 9
ISBN 0 12 302558 3

I INTRODUCTION

The purpose of this article is to consider how interferon α and β species (IFNs) may function as endogenously produced physiological regulators of cellular processes in the body. The early findings that IFNs can inhibit cell proliferation in culture (Paucker *et al.*, 1962) and tumour growth in the whole organism (Gresser *et al.*, 1969) showed that their ability to inhibit viral replication was but one facet of their complex action (Gresser, 1977). The IFN system was likened to a polypeptide hormone system (Baron, 1967). The immunomodulatory capabilities of IFNs were recognized as were the complex effects of IFNs on cell differentiation (reviewed in De Mayer-Guignard and De Mayer, 1985; and in Rossi, 1985). It became evident that IFNs specifically induce numerous proteins, including several enzymes and histocompatibility antigens (reviewed in Lengyel, 1982; and Revel, 1984).

Given the wide range of effects of IFNs on cell proliferation, differentiation, and tumour growth, attention is now focusing on interactions of IFNs with the burgeoning number of cell growth factors, differentiation factors, and various other cytokines, and on the ability of IFNs to suppress the expression of oncogenes. We will discuss what IFNs can do, how they may accomplish what they can do, and how they fit in among other factors with cytomodulatory actions. While focusing on systems where most information is available, we will make certain that the variety of IFN actions is continually kept in mind. Although we will not address the mechanism or broad significance of the antiviral action of IFNs, we note that the antiviral assay for IFNs is a key tool for the detection of IFNs and the analysis of their role in mediating the action of other cytokines.

We have chosen to consider IFN-α and IFN-β species collectively; however, we will pay special attention to evidence of profound differences in the inducibility of the different IFN-α and IFN-β species, and of differences in their actions. We will make comparative observations on IFN-γ in discussing IFN effects on cell differentiation and the synthesis of class I and class II major histocompatibility complex (MHC) antigens, and some other topics. IFN-α and -β species can be produced by many different cell types and in response to a wide variety of stimuli. At least some IFN-α and -β species also *appear* to be constitutively expressed. Evidence is mounting that distinct IFNs are induced under different physiological and pathological conditions, with the different IFNs playing specialized roles in the growth, development and maintenance of the organism and in defence mechanisms against disease. We will explore the question of what the physiological inducers of endogenous IFNs are.

Abbreviations: MHC, major histocompatibility complex, H-2 in the mouse, HLA in man; BSF-2, human B cell maturation (differentiation) factor; SmC (IGF-1), somatomedin C (insulin-like growth factor 1); EBV, Epstein-Barr virus; TNF, tumour necrosis factor; TPA, 12-*O*-tetradecanoyl-phorbol-13-acetate; IL, interleukin; LT, lymphotoxin; DiC_8, 1,2-dioctanoylglycerol; OAG, 1-oleoyl-1-acetylglycerol; CSF-1, colony stimulating factor 1.

Recently, evidence has been obtained that cell growth factors greatly enhance the expression of the IFN-β_2 gene, and that the IFN-β_2 produced can have a negative feedback effect on the cell growth stimulation by these factors. Moreover, it has recently become apparent through cDNA cloning and sequencing of the genes for human IFN-β_2 (Haegeman *et al.*, 1986; Zilberstein *et al.*, 1986; May *et al.*, 1986) and the human B cell differentiation factor (BSF-2) (Hirano *et al.*, 1986) that they are one and the same gene (Sehgal *et al.*, 1987a). A distinct human gene that cross-hybridizes IFN-β_2 cDNA probes has been detected in DNA from several individuals and has been isolated from two different human genomic DNA libraries (Zilberstein *et al.*, 1986; Sehgal *et al.*, 1986; Sehgal and May, 1987). It has been suggested that this gene, which yields biologically active human IFN when transfected into rodent cells (Zilberstein *et al.*, 1986), be designated IFN-β_2b and the previously characterized gene be designated IFN-β_2a. RNA hybridization analyses carried out to date in different laboratories do not distinguish between transcripts derived from the IFN-β_2a or the IFN-β_2b gene, because the IFN-β_2a probes used would cross-hybridize the heterologous IFN-β_2b mRNA. We have used the general term IFN-β_2 throughout the present article and await the detailed characterization of the transcriptional products of the IFN-β_2a- and IFN-β_2b-genes.

As would be expected of a cytokine, the actions of IFNs are subject to modulation via a number of different pathways. It has also become clear that IFNs can themselves play a dual modulating role in relation to other cytokines, i.e. they can function as suppressors of the action of at least some growth factors and at the same time serve as mediators of the antiviral or cell-surface-modulating effects of the same growth factors. Knowledge of signal transduction mechanisms operating in IFN action on cells and in the actions of other cytokines is essential for a fuller understanding of the cytokine network of which IFNs form an important part. Interactions among growth factors and IFNs lead to the question of precisely how the expression of IFN genes and of genes inducible by IFNs or growth factors is regulated at the chromosomal level. Here recent nucleotide sequence analyses are beginning to provide potentially important insights.

The physiological role of IFNs can be fully understood only within the context of the whole organism. We will therefore consider some examples of what IFNs can do in the whole organism and assess the possible roles of endogenous IFNs.

II EFFECTS OF IFNs ON CELLS IN CULTURE

We will consider in some detail two examples of IFN action on cell proliferation, chosen to illustrate the ability of IFNs to suppress the expression of specific genes in cells, and the ability of an IFN to suppress the binding of a growth factor required for the proliferation of the cells. In recent articles we have summarized evidence which shows that IFNs have marked effects on the cell membrane and the associated cytoskeletal complex (Tamm *et al.*, 1984a; Pfeffer, 1987). IFN treatment of normal or transformed cells can cause a rapid decrease in the fluidity of the plasma membrane lipid bilayer (Pfeffer *et al.*, 1981; Chatterjee *et al.*, 1982) and an increase in the abundance of organized microfilaments (Pfeffer *et al.*, 1980a; Wang *et al.*, 1981; Bourgeade *et al.*, 1981; Hicks *et al.*, 1981; Brouty-Boyé *et al.*, 1981; Lin *et al.*, 1983a). A number of the IFN-induced phenotypic changes, such as the increased microfilament organization, are the direct opposite of those commonly found after neoplastic transformation of cells in culture. It should be possible in the future to integrate structural and biochemical findings that illustrate the different aspects of IFN action on cells. In this article we will focus on phenomena involving or reflecting altered gene expression.

A Inhibition of Proliferation

1 Inhibition of cell cycle activation in quiescent mouse 3T3 fibroblasts

It is well established that IFN treatment of confluent, quiescent cultures of mouse BALB/c 3T3 cells delays or blocks serum-stimulated entry of the cells into S phase (Sokawa *et al.*, 1977; Balkwill and Taylor-Papadimitriou, 1978; Lin *et al.*, 1986a). Platelet-derived growth factor (PDGF), which is present in 10% serum-supplemented medium at a concentration of 1–2 U/ml, initiates proliferation of quiescent mouse 3T3 fibroblasts by rendering the cells competent to respond to epidermal growth factor (EGF) and somatomedin C (SmC), which are required for progression to a mid-G_1 point (Pledger *et al.*, 1977; Pledger *et al.*, 1978; Leof *et al.*, 1982). Only SmC is required for progression from mid-G_1 into S phase (Leof *et al.*, 1982). Induction of competence is dependent on RNA synthesis, and once induced in cells by PDGF, competence is transferable by cytoplasts (Smith and Stiles, 1981). With PDGF added to quiescent 3T3 cells at 15 U/ml, 2–3 hours are required to render the majority of cells responsive to progression factors (Pledger *et al.*, 1977). With lower doses of PDGF a longer time is required.

PDGF transiently increases the transcription of the c-*fos* proto-oncogene (Greenberg and Ziff, 1984) and several other genes (Lau and Nathans, 1985) within a few minutes after addition. The concentration dependence and kinetics of c-*fos* gene activation correlate closely with the occupation of cell-surface PDGF receptors on 3T3 cells (Cooper *et al.*, 1982; Müller *et al.*, 1984). Activation of the c-*fos* gene is followed within a short time by increased transcription of several additional genes, including the c-*myc* proto-oncogene (Kelly *et al.*, 1983; Cochran *et al.*, 1983). Increased synthesis of the nuclear c-*fos* protein is detected within 10 minutes of PDGF addition to 3T3 cells (Kruijer *et al.*, 1984; Müller *et al.*, 1984). Enhanced synthesis of another nuclear protein of 29 kD can also be detected early in PDGF-stimulated cells (Olashaw and Pledger, 1983). The synthesis of this protein is maximal by 3 hours and declines by 5 hours after PDGF addition. In contrast, the synthesis of a 35 kD protein increases progressively during the initial 5 hours after PDGF addition (Scher *et al.*, 1983).

Coaddition of mouse IFN-α/β with PDGF suppresses the levels of c-*fos* and c-*myc* mRNAs and also those of ornithine decarboxylase and β-actin mRNAs in the stimulated mouse BALB/c 3T3 cells (Einat *et al.*, 1985a). Whereas the induction of c-*myc* mRNA by PDGF does not depend on protein synthesis, the suppression by IFN of PDGF-induced c-*myc* gene expression does at least in part depend on protein synthesis. IFN-α/β induces a series of proteins in BALB/c 3T3 cells, of which a 54 kD band and a 47.5 kD band are the most prominent (Lin *et al.*, 1985).

In quiescent BALB/c 3T3 cells to which IFN-α/β is added simultaneously with PDGF, the enhancement of the synthesis of the nuclear 29 kD protein and the 35 kD protein is markedly inhibited at 1 and 3 hours after addition of PDGF, and their synthesis remains suppressed at 5 hours (Lin *et al.*, 1986a). Addition of IFN with PDGF to quiescent cells also inhibits the PDGF-induced disaggregation of actin fibres within 1 hour (Lin *et al.*, 1985). Moreover, the PDGF-induced increase in the overall rate of cellular protein synthesis (Owen *et al.*, 1982), which reflects the activation of cells to a cycling state (Baserga, 1985), is inhibited by IFN treatment without an effect on the basal level of protein synthesis in resting cells (Lin *et al.*, 1986a). All of these results show that IFN acts rapidly to inhibit growth factor action.

The ability of IFN to inhibit entry into S phase of quiescent 3T3 cells stimulated with 10% calf serum decreases progressively as the time interval between serum stimulation and IFN addition is increased (Lin *et al.*, 1986a). There was essentially no inhibition of S phase entry when IFN addition was delayed for longer than 6 hours after stimulation (Lin *et al.*, 1986a). These findings are consistent with the time required (5–6 hours) for a majority of the cells in a population to respond successfully to PDGF present in 10% serum-supplemented medium, and support the view that IFN delays or blocks S phase entry of cells by antagonizing the action of PDGF and not that of progression factors. This conclusion is strengthened by the finding of a similar inhibition of S phase entry regardless of whether cells are first exposed to IFN and PDGF, followed by removal and refeeding with medium containing progression factors only, or exposed to IFN and PDGF continuously in the presence of progression factors (Lin *et al.*, 1986a). Moreover, IFN addition to cells arrested midway between G_0 and S phase (Stiles *et al.*, 1979) did not decrease the synthesis of a 55 kD protein induced by the addition of progression factor-supplemented complete medium, or the entry of cells into S phase (S. L. Lin and I. Tamm, unpublished). However, these findings do not completely exclude the possibility of a direct action of IFN on some EGF-induced process during the first half of the prolonged G_1 phase of the activated cells. Indeed, earlier kinetic studies had suggested that the IFN-mediated inhibition of S phase entry of serum-stimulated BALB/c 3T3 cells was due to IFN action during the middle or late G_1 phase (Sokawa *et al.*, 1977; Kimchi *et al.*, 1981).

It is of interest that pretreatment of BALB/c 3T3 cells with IFN for 48 hours neither alters the pattern of cell-associated PDGF-induced proteins nor inhibits the ability of PDGF to enhance the levels of PDGF-induced c-*myc*, JE and KC mRNAs (Tominaga and Lengyel, 1985). A possible explanation is that IFN-induced proteins that could be responsible for the inhibition of induction of PDGF-induced mRNAs may decline to basal levels in 48 hours (Einat *et al.*, 1985a). However, pretreatment of cells for 48 hours, followed by exposure to PDGF in the presence of freshly added IFN, does inhibit the accumulation of PDGF-induced secreted proteins in addition to inhibiting cell proliferation (Tominaga and Lengyel, 1985). The 35 kD species represents a secreted glycoprotein known as the major excretion protein (MEP) (Gottesman, 1978; Gottesman and Sobel, 1980; Scher *et al.*, 1983), which is constitutively produced by Kirsten sarcoma virus-transformed NIH 3T3 cells (Gottesman, 1978; Gottesman and Sobel, 1980) and has been shown to belong to a group of thiol proteases (Gal and Gottesman, 1986). Lack of accumulation of the 35 kD protein in the medium of IFN-treated cells (Tominaga and Lengyel, 1985) is at least in part due to inhibition of its synthesis (Lin *et al.*, 1986a), and not entirely due to an inhibition of secretion, although IFN inhibits the secretion of at least one protein, i.e. plasminogen activator (Schroder *et al.*, 1978).

The products of the c-*fos*, c-*myc* and other genes induced by PDGF could all co-operate in some common cellular response or they could each mediate a different biological response (Kruijer *et al.*, 1984). The nuclear localization of the c-*fos*, c-*myc*, and the 29 kD proteins is consistent with a nuclear function. The fact that elevated levels of the c-*fos* and c-*myc* RNAs persist only for a short time, but are both superinducible by cycloheximide (Kelly *et al.*, 1983; Müller *et al.*, 1984), suggests that their expression is closely regulated. Although a high level of c-*fos* gene expression appears to be a characteristic of growth factor-induced transition from the G_0 to G_1 phase, it is not a characteristic of exponentially proliferating fibroblasts in culture (Müller *et al.*, 1984). Moreover, c-*fos* may be involved in the induction of differentiation in particular cell types (reviewed in Müller *et al.*, 1984). These findings notwithstanding, evidence has been obtained that inducible production of c-*fos* antisense RNA inhibits 3T3 cell proliferation (Holt *et al.*, 1986).

There is also evidence for a functional role for c-*myc* in the mitogenic response to PDGF, as in 3T3 subline constructs, in which hydrocortisone is the primary determinant of *myc* mRNA content, the c-*myc* gene governs clonal growth in PDGF-free medium (Armelin *et al.*, 1984). Expression of c-*myc* in such 3T3 cell sublines is, however, not associated with all of the phenotypic changes that PDGF itself induces, and only a relatively small fraction of the cells replicate DNA in a 24-hour period. Some additional evidence for a role of c-*myc* as a competence factor has been obtained in experiments in which c-*myc* protein was microinjected into nuclei of quiescent 3T3 cells (Kaczmarek *et al*, 1985). In human fibroblasts, enhanced c-*myc* expression is a common response to a diverse group of agents that elicit phosphoinositide turnover and activate protein kinase C, and is not sufficient to explain the mitogenic action of PDGF (Coughlin *et al.*, 1985). Although the c-*myc* product may be one of the mediators of the growth response to PDGF, it does not appear to be the only or the sufficient one.

It appears plausible that inhibition of the expression of PDGF-inducible genes may be one mechanism whereby IFN delays or blocks the traverse of quiescent cells from G_0/G_1 to S phase; however, it is not clear that this is the only mechanism. Moreover, to understand the molecular mechanism of IFN action on the synthesis of PDGF-inducible proteins, the total complement of such proteins needs to be precisely defined, and those proteins identified that are required to render cells competent to respond to progression factors such as EGF and SmC.

2 *Inhibition of proliferation of exponentially dividing human lymphoblastoid cells*

Exponentially growing cells of the Burkitt's lymphoma lines P_3HR-1 (Leandersson and Lundgren, 1980, 1982) or Daudi (Einat *et al.*, 1985b) become arrested in the G_0/G_1 phase after treatment with IFN-α. The process of identifying those IFN-induced events that may be causally related to the cessation of cell proliferation is aided by the availability of cloned IFN-resistant mutant sublines of Daudi cells (such as DIF_2 and DIF_3 (Dron and Tovey, 1983; Tovey *et al.*, 1983). These IFN-resistant sublines of Daudi cells possess high-affinity IFN receptors in numbers (approximately 3000) similar to the numbers of such receptors on the surface of IFN-sensitive parent Daudi cells (Tovey *et al.*, 1983; Pfeffer *et al.*, 1986, 1987a), and, like parent cells, they respond to IFN with increased production of 2′,5′A synthetase (Dron and Tovey, 1983; Tovey *et al.*, 1983). Nevertheless, there are striking differences in the complements of proteins induced by IFN-α in the sensitive and resistant cells (Dron *et al.*, 1985). Of the 15 proteins induced by IFN in parental cells, only eight could be detected in IFN-resistant clones of Daudi cells, and, among these eight, some appeared later and in smaller amounts than in IFN-treated parental cells. Moreover, IFN-α inhibits the synthesis of the heavy μ-chains of IgM in a clone of IFN-sensitive Daudi cells, but not in Daudi cells that are resistant to the anti-growth action of IFN, although IFN induces the double-stranded RNA-dependent protein kinase and 2′,5′A synthetase in the resistant cells. IFN-sensitive cells treated with IFN show decreased levels of μ-chain mRNA (Hovanessian *et al.*, 1986). No differences have been detected in the complements of constitutive proteins present in resistant sublines versus parental Daudi cells (Dron *et al.*, 1985).

Insulin and transferrin receptors. The proliferation of both IFN-sensitive and IFN-resistant Daudi cells can be regulated by two factors: insulin and transferrin (Pfeffer *et al.*, 1986). Proliferation of both kinds of Daudi cells is dependent on occupancy of insulin receptors, with the most rapid proliferation occurring at close to 100% receptor occupancy. Daudi cells lack receptors for insulin-like growth-factor I (Pfeffer *et al.*, 1986, 1987b). IFN treatment decreases the capacity of IFN-sensitive cells to bind insulin (Pfeffer *et al.*, 1986). This is due to a decrease in lower affinity insulin-binding sites ($K_d = 6.3$ nM) on the cell surface. In contrast, IFN treatment of IFN-resistant cells has no effect on their insulin-binding capacity. Higher affinity insulin binding ($K_d = 0.01$ nM) to either sensitive or resistant cells is not altered by IFN treatment. Insulin binding is also reduced in detergent-solubilized extracts from IFN-treated sensitive Daudi cells, and the magnitude of the decrease is comparable to that observed in intact cells. Thus, the total number of insulin binding sites (surface and internal) appears to be decreased in IFN-treated sensitive Daudi cells (Pfeffer *et al.*, 1986, 1987b). It may be noted that murine IFN-γ did not affect insulin binding to 3T3-L1 cells which had differentiated into adipocytes (Patton *et al.*, 1986).

The fact that the proliferation of Daudi cells is directly related to insulin concentration in the range (10^{-10}–10^{-7} M), in which binding is primarily of the lower affinity type, strongly supports the view that lower affinity insulin binding is important for the growth of Daudi cells. If this is so, then the ability of IFN to decrease lower affinity insulin binding in IFN-sensitive cells is likely to be causally related to the antiproliferative effect of IFN on these cells. Following IFN addition to IFN-sensitive cells, lower affinity insulin binding decreases linearly with time between 6 and 48 hours. The effect of IFN on lower affinity insulin binding sites is more rapid than that on cell proliferation (Pfeffer *et al.*, 1987b). This kinetic evidence is also consistent with the possibility that decreased binding of the surface of IFN-treated cells may be one of the factors responsible for the inhibitory effect of IFN on Daudi cell proliferation (Pfeffer *et al.*, 1987b).

There is a clear distinction between the regulation of the insulin and transferrin receptors. The number of insulin receptors is similar in exponentially dividing and plateau phase cells (Pfeffer *et al.*, 1987b), whereas the number of transferrin receptors is greater in exponentially dividing cells (Larrick and Creswell, 1979). Upon feeding of plateau phase cells, the number of transferrin receptors increases (Besançon *et al.*, 1985), but the number of insulin receptors remain stable (Pfeffer *et al.*, 1987b). IFN-α largely blocks the increase in the number of transferrin receptors which occurs upon feeding of plateau phase Daudi cells (Besançon *et al.*, 1985). Since low transferrin receptor levels are associated with G_1 phase cells (Musgrove *et al.*, 1984), and since IFN treatment arrests lymphoblastoid cells in the G_0/G_1 phase (Leandersson and Lundgren, 1980, 1982; Einat *et al.*, 1985b), such an effect would be expected. Of interest is the finding that IFN-α down-regulates transferrin receptors on IFN-sensitive, but not on IFN-resistant, Daudi cells (Pfeffer *et al.*, 1987b).

It has been reported that human IFN-α_2 inhibits the binding of EGF to Madin-Darby bovine kidney cells (MDBK), and the proliferation of these cells (Zoon *et al.*, 1986a). The decreased binding of EGF to IFN-α_2-treated cells appears to reflect both a down-regulation of the number of EGF receptors and a reduction in the affinity of EGF for its receptors. IFN-β and -γ have little effect on EGF binding and proliferation of MDBK cells (Zoon *et al.*, 1986a). It is not clear whether EGF stimulates the proliferation of MDBK cells, what the effect was of a significant fraction (15%) of the ligand being acid-soluble, and why, based on acid resistance, a substantial fraction (25%) of the bound EGF appears to have been internalized at 4° (Zoon *et al.*, 1986a). In earlier experiments (Lin *et al.*, 1980) IFN-β was found to inhibit EGF-stimulated uptake of thymidine into DNA in human fibroblasts without affecting EGF binding to cells.

c-myc proto-oncogene. IFN-β causes a marked selective reduction in steady state c-*myc* mRNA levels in Daudi cells within 3 hours (Jonak and Knight, 1984; Dani *et al.*, 1985). Nuclear run-on experiments that measured the rate of transcription across the second exon of c-*myc* did not reveal a significant effect of IFN-β on c-*myc* transcription in this region, which led to the suggestion that IFN-β may regulate the expression of c-*myc* mRNA at a post-transcriptional level (Knight *et al.*, 1985).

IFN-α also causes a two- to several-fold reduction in c-*myc* mRNA in Daudi cells (Einat *et al.*, 1985b; Dani *et al.*, 1985; Dron *et al.*, 1986). In one laboratory (Dani *et al.*, 1985), nuclear run-on experiments that measured the rate of transcription across the first c-*myc* exon or across both the second and third exons did not yield evidence of a decreased rate of c-*myc* gene transcription, and actinomycin D chase experiments indicated a marked reduction in the half-life of c-*myc* RNA in IFN-α treated cells (Dani *et al.*,

1985). However, in another laboratory (Einat *et al.*, 1985b), nuclear run-on experiments that measured the rate of transcription across the third exon of c-*myc* indicated that IFN-α treatment decreased the rate of c-*myc* gene transcription in this region. IFN treatment of a Daudi cell variant that is resistant to the antiproliferative effect of IFN does not cause a decrease in c-*myc* mRNA, and the cells do not become arrested in G_0/G_1, although they do make increased amounts of 2′,5′A synthetase, as do sensitive cells (Einat *et al.*, 1985b; Dron *et al.*, 1986). IFN treatment did not significantly affect c-*myc* expression in a clone of IFN-resistant cells which had reverted to almost full sensitivity to the antiproliferative action of IFN (Dron *et al.*, 1986). Thus, a reduced level of c-*myc* mRNA may not be a prerequisite for inhibition of cell proliferation in IFN-treated cells. It is also of interest that in human HeLa cells, IFN-α causes a two-fold decrease in the c-*myc* mRNA level, whereas IFN-γ causes a three-fold increase, although the inhibition of cell growth is greater with IFN-γ (Kelly *et al.*, 1985).

In Daudi cells the c-*myc* gene has become transcriptionally highly active through a specific chromosomal translocation (Erikson *et al.*, 1983). The most common form of this translocation involves a break in the c-*myc* gene between the first and second exons and places the second and third exons within an immunoglobulin locus (Leder *et al.*, 1983). Thus, the second exon, which contains the initiating ATG codon, represents the promoter-proximal region of the rearranged c-*myc* gene. It has been shown recently that the promoter-proximal region of the murine c-*myc* gene is transcribed in Friend erythroleukaemia cells at a molarity that far exceeds transcription through the rest of the gene (Mechti *et al.*, 1986). When Friend cells are induced to differentiate by DMSO, transcription through the c-*myc* gene is blocked some distance from the promoter, so that the promoter-proximal region continues to be transcribed at a high rate whereas the promoter-distal transcription is strongly inhibited (Mechti *et al.*, 1986). This effect is strongly reminiscent of the mechanism by which 5,6-dichloro-1-β-D-ribofuranosyl-benzimidazole (DRB) blocks RNA transcription in mammalian cells (Sehgal *et al.*, 1976, 1979; Fraser *et al.*, 1978, 1979; Tamm, 1977; Tamm and Kikuchi, 1979; Tamm *et al.*, 1980; reviewed in Tamm *et al.* 1984c). DRB blocks transcription by enhancing the premature termination (attenuation) of RNA several hundred nucleotides from the promoter. In the studies of Knight *et al.* (1985) and Dani *et al.* (1985), RNA transcription across the promoter-distal third exon of c-*myc* was not measured, whereas transcription across this region was investigated by Einat *et al.* (1985b). It is possible that the inhibitory effect of IFNs on transcription across the rearranged c-*myc* gene in Daudi cells is like that of DRB i.e., transcription across the promoter-proximal region continues unaffected but that across the promoter-distal region is strongly inhibited.

In normal lymphocytes and fibroblasts the c-*myc* gene is regulated by cell growth-stimulating agents in a cell cycle-dependent manner (Kelly *et al.*, 1983). The specific induction of the c-*myc* gene expression in normal human B cells is, however, not itself a sufficient event for acquisition of competence to proliferate (Smeland *et al.*, 1985). Additional inducible functions appear to be needed to potentiate the *myc*-specific function in order for the B cells to acquire the capacity to proliferate in response to the B cell growth factor.

From kinetic evidence, it does not appear likely that decreased expression of the c-*myc* gene after IFN treatment is secondary to the down-regulation of insulin receptors. Nor is there evidence that the abundance of insulin receptors is dependent on c-*myc* expression, or that the IFN-caused decrease in the number of insulin receptors is mediated via decreased c-*myc* expression. It appears at present that the decreased insulin binding by IFN-sensitive cells is likely to be at least in part responsible for the decreased proliferation of the IFN-treated cells. Whether decreased c-*myc* expression plays a similar role is less clear.

Recombinant human IFN-α and -γ species have been compared with respect to their ability to inhibit the proliferation of normal B lymphocytes infected *in vitro* with Epstein-Barr virus (EBV) and tumour-derived cell lines (Torsteindottir *et al.*, 1985). EBV-induced B-cell proliferation is highly sensitive to inhibition by IFN-α and less sensitive to IFN-γ. IFN-α inhibits the proliferation of three Burkitt lymphoma-derived cell lines, Raji, Daudi, and Namalwa, when the cells are propagated either in suspension or clonogenically in semisolid medium, with each cell line displaying a characteristic sensitivity. Although IFN-γ has no effect on proliferation in suspension, it abolishes the clonogenic potential of the tumour cell lines in semisolid agarose. These results highlight the complexity of IFN effects on cells. The clonogenic assay provides a means of evaluating IFN action on tumour cells that can be useful in patient selection for therapy (Strayer *et al.*, 1984).

B Enhancement or Inhibition of Differentiation

As recently summarized and discussed by Rossi (1985), IFNs affect the differentiation of many types of cells, and the effects of IFNs on cell differentiation are generally reversible once IFN is removed. Most of those examples of the ability of IFNs to enhance or inhibit differentiation which we will consider have been published since Rossi's review. An important development in the field is the recognition that human IFN-β_2 and B cell differentiation factor (BSF-2), whose genes have been independently cloned and sequenced (Haegeman *et al.*, 1986; Zilberstein *et al.*, 1986; May *et al.*, 1986; Hirano *et al.*, 1986), represent one and the same cytokine (Sehgal *et al.*,

1987a). BSF-2 induces antibody production and secretion by activated B lymphocytes (reviewed in Kishimoto, 1985; Kikutani *et al.*, 1985; Hirano *et al.*, 1985; Hirano *et al.*, 1986). Human IFN-β_2 (Sehgal and Sagar, 1980; Weissenbach *et al.*, 1980; Sagar *et al.*, 1982; reviewed in Sehgal, 1982; Sehgal *et al.*, 1986; Kohase *et al.*, 1986, 1987a; Haegeman *et al.*, 1986; Zilberstein *et al.*, 1986; May *et al.*, 1986) is characteristically induced in quiescent human fibroblasts by mitogenic stimulation with, e.g., tumour necrosis factor (TNF), and then suppresses the mitogenic effect of the stimulating agent (Kohase *et al.*, 1986). The antimitogenic activity of recombinant IFN-β_2 in human fibroblasts is 10 times higher, on an antiviral unit basis, than that of IFN-β_1 (cited in Revel and Zilberstein, 1987). IFN-β_2/BSF-2 is identical with a human protein that stimulates the growth of certain murine hybridoma and plasmacytoma cell lines ("hybridoma growth factor") (Van Damme *et al.*, 1987).

IFN-β_2/BSF-2 induces an increase in the level of mRNA specific for secretory heavy chains and then induces the final maturation of B cells into immunoglobulin-secreting cells (Kikutani *et al.*, 1985). Earlier work had shown that IFN-β_2/BSF-2 induces IgM and IgG secretion in *Staphylococcus aureus*-activated normal B cells (Okada *et al.*, 1983; Teranishi *et al.*, 1984) and in EBV-transformed human B cell lines (Muraguchi *et al.*, 1981; Teranishi *et al.*, 1982). The induction of antibody secretion by IFN-β_2/BSF-2 in EBV-transformed B cells was not associated with any effect on cell growth. In contrast, IFN-α inhibits the synthesis of the μ-chains of IgM in Daudi cells and the proliferation of Daudi cells (Hovanessian *et al.*, 1986).

IFN-β_2/BSF-2 is produced not only by helper T cells, but also by human fibroblasts (Poupart *et al.*, 1984; Kohase *et al.*, 1986, 1987a), human monocytes/macrophages (Vaquero *et al.*, 1986), in certain T cell lines (Hirano *et al.*, 1986), in T24 bladder carcinoma cells (Hirano *et al.*, 1986; Wong and Goeddel, 1986), in cardiac myxoma cells (Hirano *et al.*, 1986) and probably by a variety of other cells. In human lymphocytes, the expression of IFN-β_2/BSF-2 can be enhanced by 12-*O*-tetradecanoyl-phorbol-13-acetate (TPA) (Hirano *et al.*, 1986). In human diploid fibroblasts, its expression is enhanced by TNF, interleukin-1 (IL-1), lymphotoxin (LT), PDGF, IFN-α, -β, and -γ, and poly(I).poly(C) (Content *et al.*, 1985; Kohase *et al.*, 1986, 1987a; May *et al.*, 1986; Wong and Goeddel, 1986). 1,2-Dioctanoylglycerol (DiC_8) and 1-oleoyl-2-acetylglycerol (OAG) also strongly increase IFN-β_2/BSF-2 expression in human fibroblasts (Sehgal *et al.*, 1987a,b).

IFN-α, -β, and -γ all induced blast transformation and plasmacytoid differentiation with intracellular Ig expression in leukaemic B cells from 19 of 29 patients with chronic B lymphocytic leukaemia (Östlund *et al.*, 1986). IFN-α, -β, and -γ gave rise to a proliferative response by the leukaemic B cells from 3 of the 29 patients. It is possible that endogenous production of

IFN-β_2/BSF-2 in IFN-treated cells (Kohase *et al.*, 1987a) is involved in these phenomena.

IFN-α and -γ can act as cytotoxic T lymphocyte differentiation signals (Chen *et al.*, 1986a, b). Human T cell clones that are able to proliferate in response to specific stimuli, but cannot kill even in the presence of lectins, acquire the specific lytic function when exposed to recombinant IFN-α or -γ (Chen *et al.*, 1986a). Coincident with the acquisition of cytotoxic function, IFN-α appears to induce a rearrangement in the gene for the T cell receptor α-chain (Chen *et al.*, 1986b). Furthermore, in a mature clone of cytotoxic T lymphocytes, which already shows lytic function and in which this gene is already rearranged, IFN-α appears to induce a new arrangement of the gene for the T cell receptor α-chain (Chen *et al.*, 1986b).

IFN-α inhibits the proliferation of the human promyelocytic leukaemic cell line HL-60 without inducing differentiation (Grant *et al.*, 1985). When IFN-α is combined with differentiation-inducing agents such as TPA, retinoic acid or dimethyl sulphoxide, growth suppression and induction of differentiation are greatly increased. IFN-γ does, however, itself induce differentiation of human promyelocytic cell lines along the monocytic pathway, as indicated by co-ordinate expression of monocyte markers and functions such as monocyte-specific surface antigens, class II HLA-DR antigens, nonspecific esterase, receptors for the Fc fragment of IgG, and the ability to mediate antibody-dependent cell-mediated cytotoxicity (Dayton *et al.*, 1985). Differentiation induced by IFN-γ does not appear to be secondary to an arrest of growth of promyelocytic cells. The differentiation activity of conditioned medium from lectin-stimulated human leukocytes is due to the synergistic effect of IFN-γ and other factors which have not yet been identified (Dayton *et al.*, 1985).

The effects of IFN-α on the *in vitro* differentiation of human blood monocytes into macrophages are complex and dose-dependent (Hovi *et al.*, 1985). At higher concentrations, almost all of the cells remain small and rounded. At lower concentrations of IFN, bipolar spreading of cells takes place with the result that most monocytes become elongated fibroblastoid cells (Hovi *et al.*, 1985). In this system IFN inhibits, in a dose-dependent manner, the formation of actin- and vinculin-containing adhesion plaques, which play a role in mediating adherence of human monocytes to the growth substratum. The effect of IFN on the adhesion plaques may be secondary to primary effects on the commitment process to differentiation.

Mouse IFN causes a concentration-dependent inhibition of both spontaneous and melanocyte hormone-stimulated melanogenesis in cultures of murine B-16 melanoma cells, with a concomitant inhibition of tyrosinase activity (Fisher *et al.*, 1981). Different human melanoma cell lines vary in their sensitivity to the growth-inhibitory effects of recombinant IFN-β, but

IFN-β is more active than recombinant IFN-α species (Fisher *et al.*, 1985). The cell lines also vary in their sensitivity to the cell growth-inhibitory effect of the antileukaemic compound mezerein, which shares a number of properties with phorbol esters, including the ability to modulate differentiation (Fisher *et al.*, 1985). The combination of IFN-β and mezerein caused a more marked inhibition of proliferation of all four melanoma cell lines, and resulted in higher levels of melanin than those observed with either agent alone.

IFN also inhibits the differentiation of chicken embryo myogenic cells, as measured by creatine kinase isoenzyme transition and myotube formation (Grossberg and Sabran, 1982; Lough *et al.*, 1982; Tomida and Hasegawa, 1984), and the differentiation in a murine myoblast line (MM14D2), as indicated by a dose-dependent reduction of myotube formation and creatine kinase activity (Multhauf and Lough, 1986). Increases in DNA content suggested that the myoblasts whose differentiation was inhibited continued to proliferate (Multhauf and Lough, 1986). The murine IFN-β-treated myoblasts maintained ornithine decarboxylase activity at control levels, and exogenous polyamines did not prevent the inhibitory effect of IFN on differentiation. Thus, IFN action was not mediated via the polyamine pathway, the products of which are required for myogenesis. In contrast, Hu-rIFN-αA causes an acceleration of myotube formation and creatine kinase isoenzyme transition from CK-BB to CK-MM in normal human myoblast cultures derived from mature skeletal muscle (Fisher *et al.*, 1983). Differences in the results may reflect differences in the systems or IFNs used or both.

IFN inhibits the adipose conversion of BALB/c (Cioé *et al.*, 1980) and insulin-stimulated 3T3-L1 cells (Keay and Grossberg, 1980). In the insulin-stimulated 3T3-L1 cells, IFN treatment decreases the rate of synthesis and accumulation of triglycerides, cholesterol esters, and cholesterol, and prevents the loss of submembranous cytoskeletal filaments (Keay and Grossberg, 1980; Grossberg and Keay, 1980). The protein profile of cells treated with IFN and insulin resembles the profile of control cells (Keay and Grossberg, 1980; Grossberg and Sabran, 1982). As mentioned above, the insulin-binding capacity of IFN-treated 3T3-L1 adipocytes is unchanged (Patton *et al.*, 1986).

Recombinant murine IFN-γ, human hybrid IFN-α_2/α_1, and human TNF and LT all inhibit [^{3}H] acetate uptake by adipocytes derived from 3T3-L1 cells, acetate incorporation into both membrane and storage lipids, and herapin-releasable lipoprotein lipase activity (Patton *et al.*, 1986). These cytokines also suppress acetate uptake in 3T3-L1 fibroblasts, but to a lesser degree. Preexposure of adipocytes or fibroblasts to γ-IFN enhances the binding of TNF to its receptors (Patton *et al.*, 1986).

In human HeLa-S3 tumour cells, IFN-β has selective effects on lipid metabolism (Pfeffer *et al.*, 1985). IFN treatment decreases acetate incorporation into cholesterol esters, but increases incorporation into cholesterol and phosphatidylcholine, while having no effect on incorporation into sphingomyelin or phosphatidylethanolamine, as measured by continuous labelling with [^{14}C]acetate. IFN increases cholesterol synthesis measured by 1 hour pulse-labelling with [^{3}H]acetate. The finding of increased synthesis is consistent with a model according to which IFN-β treatment of HeLa cells inhibits the endocytosis of cholesterol-containing low-density lipoprotein, which results in up-regulation of cholesterol synthesis (Pfeffer *et al.*, 1985).

Recent studies have shown that human IFN-α and -β species inhibit the proliferation and differentiation of human keratinocytes in culture (Yaar *et al.*, 1985; Stadler *et al.*, 1986). Differentiation was assessed by the desquamation rate of cells from the colony surface and by the proportion of cells having cornified envelopes (Yaar *et al.*, 1985), or by polyacrylamide gel electrophoresis of six specific protein fractions to determine the amount and synthesis of non-covalently bound keratins versus disulphide crosslinked keratins (Stadler *et al.*, 1986). Yaar *et al.* (1985) found that IFN effects on both growth and differentiation are reversible within days of its removal from the medium.

In a number of cell systems the induction of differentiation by chemical means (e.g. dimethyl sulphoxide in Friend leukaemia cells) or by natural inducers (e.g. lung-conditioned medium in M1 myeloid cells) is associated with endogenous production of IFN. We will discuss these findings in Section III-A.

C Inhibition of Transformation

In Section II-A, evidence was summarized showing that IFN treatment can suppress the expression of a number of cellular proto-oncogenes under conditions in which IFN-treated cells remain or become arrested in G_0/G_1. IFNs can also suppress oncogene expression in transformed cells.

Treatment of Rous sarcoma virus-transformed rat cells (RR1022) with rat IFN-α decreases the intracellular pp60^{src}-associated protein kinase activity (Lin *et al.*, 1983a). The RR1022 cell line is derived from a fibrosarcoma induced by the Schmidt-Ruppin strain of Rous sarcoma virus, and expresses plasma membrane-associated pp60^{src}, the transforming gene product of Rous sarcoma virus. The IFN-caused decrease in pp60^{src} tyrosine kinase is due to selective inhibition of the synthesis of pp60^{src} (Lin *et al.*, 1983a), which in turn appears to reflect a decreased content of pp60^{src} mRNA (S. L. Lin and I.

Tamm, 1984, unpublished data). IFN treatment did not alter the phosphopeptide pattern of immunoprecipitated $pp60^{src}$ determined after cleavage with *S. aureus* V8 protease. A decrease in the growth rate of IFN-treated Rous sarcoma virus-transformed cells was accompanied by increases in the thickness and number of actin fibres per cell (Lin *et al.*, 1983a).

Human bladder carcinoma cell line RT4 expresses the c-*ras* proto-oncogene, the product of which is a protein doublet of approximately 21 kD (Der and Cooper, 1983). RT4 cells treated with IFN-β at cell growth inhibitory concentrations showed, as the most prominent finding, reduced levels of phosphorylated 40 and 60 kD proteins after labelling of cell extracts with γ-labelled [^{32}P]ATP or [^{32}P]GTP (Soslau *et al.*, 1984). IFN treatment of cells also resulted in decreased *in vitro* phosphorylation of 22 and 23.5 kD proteins with a concomitant increase in phosphorylation of 23 and 24.5 kD proteins. Exposure of cells to IFN decreased the amount of mRNA hybridizable with *src*-Rous and *ras*-Harvey cDNA probes without causing a reduction in *ras*-Kirsten-hybridizable mRNA, suggesting that the IFN-induced reduction of p60 and p21 results from transcriptional control of specific oncogenes, notably *src* and *ras* (Soslau *et al.*, 1984). However, the 21 kD *ras* product has not been shown to be a phosphoprotein in human cells (Der and Cooper, 1983), although similar proteins in lower animals are phosphorylated (Furth *et al.*, 1982).

A line of NIH 3T3 cells (RS 485), transformed by the human c-HA-*ras*I proto-oncogene activated by Ha-MuSV long terminal repeats, undergoes IFN-induced phenotypic reversion (Samid *et al.*, 1984, 1985). When RS 485 cells are grown in the presence of mouse IFN for 10 to 20 population doublings, flat colonies of contact-inhibited cells appear. The revertant cells, which are unable to grow in soft agar, contain the transfected oncogenic DNA in undiminished quantity and unchanged distribution as compared to parental RS 485 cells. The Ha-*ras* mRNA content is, however, decreased four-fold in the revertant cells without detectable reduction in collagen and actin mRNAs. Furthermore, the c-Ha-*ras*I gene-encoded 21 kD protein is also decreased four-fold in the revertant clones (Samid *et al.*, 1984, 1985).

Reversion of BALB/c embryonic fibroblasts, transformed by Moloney sarcoma virus, has been obtained by cultivation for over 600 generations in the presence of mouse IFN-α/β (Sergiescu *et al.*, 1986). The *mos* oncogene, whose product is cytoplasmic, acquires strong oncogenicity when linked to a constitutive promoter (Blair, *et al.*, 1981; reviewed in Weinberg, 1985). These phenotypically normal revertant cells are unable to produce tumours in nude mice, in spite of the fact that the revertant cell DNA contains at least twice as many copies of the v-*mos* oncogene as well as additional integration sites as compared to DNA from transformed cells not cultivated with IFN (Sergiescu *et al.*, 1986). Polyadenylated RNA from both revertant and control cells contains two *mos*-specific transcripts, but only control cells produce virus, while both produce helper virus. This suggests that there is a selective post-transcriptional block in v-*mos* gene expression in the revertant cells. After culture of the revertant cells for 100 additional passages in the absence of IFN, the cells still maintain their non-tumorigenic character in spite of the persistent transcription of the v-*mos* oncogene.

Examination of IFN action in simian virus 40-transformed cells superinfected with simian virus 40 has shown that, even within the same cell, the IFN system can discriminate between expression of the T antigen gene in the SV40 viral genome and expression of the same gene integrated into a host chromosome (Garcia-Blanco *et al.*, 1985). These results confirm and extend a series of previous studies (Metz *et al.*, 1976; Mozes and Defendi, 1979; Brennan and Stark, 1983) showing that IFN can inhibit the expression of one and the same gene in the viral but not in the host cell genome.

Human adenovirus 12-transformed murine cells express the class I H-2 antigens at greatly reduced levels and are highly tumorigenic in syngeneic hosts (Hayashi *et al.*, 1985). A brief treatment of the transformed cells with murine IFN-α/β or -γ causes a rapid but transient increase in the expression of class I H-2 antigens, which is accompanied by a reduction in tumorigenicity in immunocompetent hosts. The significance of these findings is not clear, because detailed studies with numerous adenovirus 2- or adenovirus 5-transformed hamster and mouse lines have revealed no correlation between tumorigenicity in immunocompetent syngeneic rodents and the level of expression of class I H-2 antigens on the surface of the transformed cells (Haddada *et al.*, 1986). However, adenovirus 12 is oncogenic, whereas adenovirus serotypes 2 and 5 are non-oncogenic, which may explain the seemingly contradictory results obtained in the above studies. Human IFN-γ is capable of restoring the synthesis of class I HLA antigens in transformed human cells that produce adenovirus 12 E1A proteins (Vasavada *et al.*, 1986). The E1A gene can greatly reduce the levels of class I HLA mRNA and antigens in the absence of E1B genes. This is noteworthy because the 1A early protein of adenovirus, like the immediate early protein of herpes virus, has the ability to increase transcription from a variety of genes by seemingly being able to eliminate the need of some genes for enhancer elements (Darnell *et al.*, 1986). It is possible that the product of one of these genes is capable of suppressing class I HLA gene expression. Infection with herpes simplex virus 1 (HSV-1) or 2 (HSV-2) suppresses the expression of the class I H-2 antigens on the surface of murine cells, with HSV-2 infection having a much greater effect (Jennings *et al.*, 1985). This may be a factor contributing to reduced lysis of HSV-2-infected cells by cytotoxic lymphocytes.

Normal rat kidney cells infected by the non-transforming Moloney murine leukaemia virus become susceptible to transformation by chemical carcinogens (Hassan *et al.*, 1985). When cells are exposed to a chemical carcinogen at a low subculture passage post-infection, under which condition transformation is detectable only after many subsequent passages, mouse IFN inhibits transformation by the carcinogen. The inhibitory effect of IFN is reversible upon removal of IFN even after the cells have been passaged many times in the presence of IFN. The inhibition of transformation by IFN is not associated with detectable effects on the proliferation or focus-forming capacity of the cells (Hassan *et al.*, 1985).

Serial passage for extended periods of time of three tumour cell lines derived from human colon, urinary bladder, and ovarian carcinoma in the continuous presence of human IFN-α gave rise to phenotypic changes that differed among the cell lines (Brouty-Boyé *et al.*, 1985). IFN-α enhanced aggregation of colon tumour cells but inhibited that of bladder tumour cells. IFN-α inhibited the proliferation of bladder and ovarian cells more than that of colon cells; however, the tumorigenicity of colon tumour cells injected i.p. or s.c. was markedly reduced after passage of the cells in the presence of IFN, while that of bladder tumour cells was not affected. The tumorigenicity of IFN-treated ovarian tumour cells was reduced when these cells were injected i.p., but not when they were injected s.c.

That IFN-induced phenotypic changes in tumour cell lines are not necessarily associated with changes in oncogene expression has been illustrated by studies in which human osteosarcoma (OHA) cells, bladder carcinoma (EJ) cells, and gastric sarcoma (SHAC) cells were passaged in the presence of IFN-α for extended periods of time (Brouty-Boyé *et al.*, 1986). OHA cells showed partial reversion of the tumour cell phenotype as exemplified by inhibition of cell proliferation, lack of cellular overlapping in confluent cultures and marked reduction in tumorigenicity for nude mice. In contrast, EJ and SHAC cells showed no reversion. In fact, passage in the presence of IFN-α resulted in potentiation of some of the phenotypic characteristics (including tumorigenicity) of SHAC cells. IFN treatment did not alter the transforming ability, gene copy number, or expression of activated oncogenes, c-Ki-*ras*, c-Ha-*ras*, and N-*ras*, respectively, in the three tumour cell lines (Brouty-Boyé *et al.*, 1986).

Transformed cells in culture commonly display a disrupted actin-containing microfilament system. IFN treatment has been shown to increase the organized state of cytoplasmic microfilaments in transformed as well as untransformed cells (Pfeffer *et al.*, 1980a; Wang *et al.*, 1981; Bourgeade *et al.*, 1981; Hicks *et al.*, 1981; Brouty-Boyé *et al.*, 1981; Lin *et al.*, 1983a). In addition, IFN treatment increases the organization and amount of cell surface fibronectin (Pfeffer *et al.*, 1980a; Bourgeade *et al.*, 1981). IFN treatment also decreases the fluidity of the plasma membrane lipid bilayer (Pfeffer *et al.*, 1981; Chatterjee *et al.*, 1982). Possibly related to these changes are the findings that IFNs can suppress both receptor-mediated endocytosis and fluid-phase pinocytosis (Pfeffer and Tamm, 1982; Whitaker-Dowling *et al.*, 1983; Wilcox *et al.*, 1983; Wang *et al.*, 1984; Lin *et al.*, 1986b) and receptor capping on the cell surface (Matsuyama, 1979; Pfeffer *et al.*, 1980b, 1986), as well as other motile functions of cells, such as translocation on a substrate (Pfeffer *et al.*, 1980a; Brouty-Boyé and Zetter, 1980). IFNs may not inhibit cell motility in all cell systems (Huygen and Verschueren, 1986).

III HOW ARE IFN EFFECTS MEDIATED?

A Signal Transduction

1 IFN receptors

The initial step in the interaction of cells with IFN is its binding to high-affinity cell surface receptors (Aguet, 1980; Branca and Baglioni, 1981). In general, the dissociation constant for IFN-α and -β is 20–500 pM and there are from several hundred to several thousand receptors per cell. The number of cell surface receptors for IFN is at least 10–100-fold lower than that reported for peptide hormones such as insulin and epidermal growth factor. Results from studies on the induction of translation-inhibitory enzymes, on transcription of IFN-inducible genes, and on the antiviral and cell growth-inhibitory actions of IFN, indicate the presence of spare receptors for IFN-α, as only a small fraction of available sites elicits maximal cellular response (Baglioni *et al.*, 1982; Hannigan and Williams, 1986; Pfeffer *et al.*, 1986). Type I IFNs (α and β) appear to share a common cell surface receptor, while type II IFN (γ) appears to bind to a separate distinct cell surface receptor (Branca and Baglioni, 1981). Other cytokines, such as lymphotoxin, IL-1 and IL-2, do not compete with IFN-α for binding to its cell surface receptors (Pfeffer, unpublished observations). Affinity cross-linking and partial purification of solubilized IFN receptor preparations has shown that the IFN-α–receptor complex is 140–150,000 M_r with a Stokes radius of $\sim$75 Å (Faltynek *et al.*, 1983; Traub *et al.*, 1984).

Although IFN binding to the cell surface is an important event, IFN binding alone is not sufficient to induce antiviral and antiproliferative activity. Several IFN-resistant cell lines have been characterized that bind amounts of IFN similar to those bound by the companion IFN-sensitive cell line. Also, IFN induces 2′,5′A synthetase and dsRNA-dependent protein kinase in both sensitive and resistant cell lines (Hovanessian *et al.*, 1986; Tovey *et al.*, 1983). After the initial interaction of IFN-α with the cell, an "activated" IFN–receptor complex is formed (Mogenson and Bandu, 1983; Pfeffer *et al.*, 1987a). Recent evidence indicates that the association of IFN–

receptor complexes with the cytoskeletal matrix is an important factor correlated with the sensitivity of Daudi lymphoblastoid cells to the antiproliferative action of IFN (Pfeffer *et al.*, 1987a). IFN-resistant Daudi cell subclones form less of a cytoskeleton-associated complex than do control cells. As with many other ligands, subsequent to the binding of cell surface receptors, IFN is internalized into the cytoplasm by the pathway of receptor-mediated endocytosis, where it is degraded, and then released from the cell (Zoon *et al.*, 1983). Treatment with the lysosomotropic amine, chloroquine, blocks the uptake, degradation, and release of degraded IFN-α but does not affect the induction of antiviral activity by IFN in Daudi cells (Branca *et al.*, 1982). Thus, internalization of IFN–receptor complexes does not appear to be an important event in IFN-α action. It has been reported that IFN-sensitive cells possess nuclear binding sites for IFNs (Kushnaryov *et al.*, 1985); however, it is not clear whether IFN binds to the nucleus under physiological conditions.

2 *Second messengers*

The Ca^{2+}-diacylglycerol messenger system and the cAMP messenger system commonly function in concert to couple stimulus to response in differentiated animal cells; however, the patterns of interaction between the two systems vary among cell types (reviewed in Rasmussen and Barrett, 1984). A discussion of the several patterns of joint regulation and control of cell functions by the two systems (see Rasmussen and Barrett, 1984; Rasmussen, 1986) is outside the scope of this article.

Binding of a cell-modulating ligand to cell surface receptors can lead to stimulation of inositol phospholipid turnover through activation of one or more phospholipase C type phosphodiesterases (reviewed in Berridge and Irvine, 1984; Berridge *et al.*, 1985; Nishizuka, 1984; Hirasawa and Nishizuka, 1985; Majerus *et al.*, 1986). As a result, phosphatidylinositol 4,5-bisphosphate is hydrolysed to noncyclic and cyclic inositol 1,4,5-trisphosphates and diacylglycerol (reviewed in Majerus *et al.*, 1986). Inositol 1,4,5-trisphosphate mediates an increase in free intracellular calcium by mobilization of Ca^{2+} from intracellular stores, which results in the activation of Ca^{2+}-calmodulin-dependent enzymes, whereas diacylglycerol activates protein kinase C. In at least some systems, signal-induced breakdown of phosphatidylinositol 4-phosphate may also occur, yielding inositol 1,4-bisophosphate and diacylglycerol, and phosphatidylinositol may be hydrolysed to inositol 1-phosphate and diacylglycerol. It is apparent that if all three inositol phospholipids are attacked by phosphodiesterases in a stimulated cell, more diacylglycerol than inositol trisphosphate will be produced, with the result that the diacylglycerol-protein kinase C-activated response is likely to be greater than the inositol trisphosphate-Ca^{2+}-activated response (Hirasawa and Nishizuka, 1985). Rapid formation of diacylglycerol can also occur from phosphatidylcholine (Daniel *et al.*, 1986; Besterman *et al.*, 1986). Diacylglycerol not only activates protein kinase C, but is also a source of arachidonic acid, a precursor of prostaglandins.

The Ca^{2+}-calmodulin and the diacylglycerol-protein kinase pathways can interact synergistically or antagonistically. In some cells in which the interaction is synergistic, the calmodulin branch may largely be responsible for the initial cellular responses and the protein kinase branch for sustained responses (reviewed in Rasmussen and Barrett, 1984; Nishizuka, 1984). The activation of protein kinase C can exert negative feedback control on calcium mobilization (see Nachshen *et al.*, 1986).

Myosin light chain kinase is a well-characterized example of a Ca^{2+}-calmodulin-activated enzyme. There are many substrates for protein kinase C, including several growth factor receptors and a ubiquitous 80 kD protein (Rozengurt *et al.*, 1983); their functions are under intensive study. Myosin light chains are phosphorylated at distinct sites by the Ca^{2+}-calmodulin-activated myosin light chain kinase and the diacylglycerol-activated protein kinase C (Nishikawa *et al.*, 1983; Naka *et al.*, 1983; Inagaki *et al.*, 1984). The 40 kD substrate for protein kinase C in platelets has been identified as inositol trisphosphate-5-phosphatase (Majerus *et al.*, 1986; Connolly *et al.*, 1986).

Binding of a ligand to cell surface receptors can also lead to stimulation of cAMP synthesis by the membrane-bound adenyl cyclase (reviewed in Rasmussen and Barrett, 1984). cAMP binds to cAMP-dependent protein kinase and thereby increases its ability to phosphorylate specific receptor proteins, such as glycogen synthase.

In addition to the above-mentioned pathways for mediating the response of cells to extracellular signals, other pathways exist. Insulin increases diacylglycerol levels without a change in the concentrations of inositol phosphates or free intracellular Ca^{2+} (Farese *et al.*, 1985). Insulin-stimulated diacylglycerol production results from the hydrolysis of a novel phosphatidylinositol-glycan (Saltiel *et al.*, 1986; Saltiel and Cuatrecasas, 1986) and this hydrolysis generates modulators of cAMP phosphodiesterase (Saltiel *et al.*, 1986).

Although many hormones are hydrophilic or large lipophilic molecules that bind to cell surface receptors, others (such as steroids) are small lipophilic molecules that diffuse through the plasma membrane and interact with cytosolic or nuclear receptors.

Human IFN-α, -β and -γ species cause a two- to three-fold increase in the concentrations of diacylglycerol within 15–30 seconds of exposure of diploid human fibroblasts to IFN (Yap *et al.*, 1986a). The concentration of diacylglycerol returns to close to the basal level within 60 seconds. In human fibroblasts, IFN-α, -β species, and IFN-γ also cause a transient rise (40–240%) in inositol trisphosphate (with IFN-β causing the greatest increase), and a smaller increase (15%) in inositol bisphosphate. The stimulatory effect of IFN-α and -β species on the diacylglycerol level is proportional to the number of IFN receptors as determined in human fibroblasts containing one, two, or three copies of chromosome 21 on which the IFN receptor gene is located. In terms of the dependence on IFN concentration, there is a correlation between the increased diacylglycerol level and antiviral effect measured with encephalomyocarditis virus.

Human Daudi lymphoblastoid cells also respond to IFN-α and -β species with a rapid increase in the diacylglycerol level (Yap *et al.*, 1986a, b). Although Daudi cells bind IFN-γ, this IFN does not induce any defined IFN effect nor increase the diacylglycerol level in these cells. In Daudi cells, the response to IFN-β is more prolonged than in fibroblasts in that after peaking at 30 seconds, the diacylglycerol level declines over the course of some minutes after IFN addition. An IFN-β concentration of 20 U/ml is sufficient to cause both a marked diacylglycerol response and a marked inhibition of Daudi cell proliferation, whereas at 200 U/ml maximal effects are obtained with respect to both parameters (Yap *et al.*, 1986b). A significant increase in diacylglycerol is demonstrable in isolated Daudi cell membranes exposed to human IFN-β (Yap *et al.*, 1986a).

In Daudi cells, IFN-β does not cause a significant increase in the concentrations of inositol bisphosphate or trisphosphate, but a transient increase in inositol monophosphate can be detected (Yap *et al.*, 1986b). No significant changes could be detected in response to IFN-β in the levels of phosphatidylinositol, phosphatidylinositol 4-phosphate, phosphatidylinositol 4,5-bisphosphate or free cytosolic Ca^{2+} (Yap *et al.*, 1986a). IFN-α also does not cause an increase in free cytosolic Ca^{2+} in Daudi cells (Nachshen *et al.*, 1986). These findings raise the question of whether IFNs increase diacylglycerol levels by increasing the hydrolysis primarily of phosphatidylinositol monophosphate, and possibly of a novel phosphatidylinositol-glycan or phosphatidylcholine, rather than of phosphatidylinositol 4,5-bisphosphate.

IFN-γ treatment of mouse peritoneal macrophages increases the protein kinase C content in these cells by as much as five-fold as determined by isolation and *in vitro* assay of the enzyme (Hamilton *et al.*, 1985). The increase was maximal 3 hours after addition of IFN-γ to cells. IFN-γ was effective at 1 U/ml, whereas IFN-α/β was ineffective even at 1000 U/ml (Hamilton *et al.*, 1985). Human IFN-β stimulates prostaglandin synthesis, possibly by promoting the release of arachidonic acid from phospholipids (Fuse *et al.*, 1982). Prednisolone and indomethacin partially inhibit the cell growth-inhibitory activity of IFN.

Measurements of cAMP levels after IFN treatment of cells have not provided strong evidence for a role for cAMP in the transduction of the IFN signal (reviewed in Tamm *et al.*, 1987). However, experiments with variant lines of macrophage-like cells of murine origin have given results suggesting that cAMP may be required for or mediate the antiproliferative action of IFN-α/β in macrophage-like cells (Schneck *et al.*, 1982).

Possible IFN effects on phosphorylation reactions that may play a role in signal transduction remain to be investigated.

B Response Molecules

Exposure of human cells to IFN can result in the activation of genes located on at least three different chromosomes: major histocompatibility complex (HLA) on chromosome 6, β_2-microglobulin on chromosome 15, and 2′,5′A synthetase on chromosome 11. Also activated are genes for several other proteins. We will focus attention on three sets of proteins, i.e., class I HLA, class II HLA, and 2′,5′A synthetase.

1 Class I HLA

Cells express HLA genes constitutively; however, IFN treatment causes a 5–10-fold increase in the mRNA for HLA-A, B, C and β_2-microglobulin in human B, T, and fibroblastic cells (Fellous *et al.*, 1982a; Burrone and Milstein, 1982; Wallach *et al.*, 1982). HLA mRNA levels increase rapidly and reach a maximum within 4 hours of IFN addition to cells; they can remain high for 24 hours (Fellous *et al.*, 1982a). The concentrations of IFN-α and -β species required to induce HLA are in the same range as those required to induce 2′,5′A synthetase and to inhibit vesicular stomatitis virus (VSV) replication. In contrast, IFN-γ induces HLA-A, B, C and β_2-microglobulin mRNAs at much lower concentrations than those required for the induction of 2′,5′A synthetase and the establishment of the antiviral state (Wallach *et al.*, 1982), as if IFN-γ had "specialized" in HLA induction (Revel, 1984). This would be consistent with the view that the immunoregulatory functions of IFN-γ may be more important than its antiviral action. Consistent with this notion are the findings that IFN-α and -β induce the synthesis of the nuclear Mx protein, which appears to block transcription of the influenza virus genome, whereas IFN-γ is unable to activate the Mx gene (Staeheli *et al.*, 1986).

The individual members of the IFN-α family differ markedly in their ability to alter the expression of a major class I HLA antigen, detected by monoclonal antibody W6/32, as well as of a number of other cell surface antigens (Greiner *et al.*, 1986). The two most potent species, IFN-αA and -αB, increased the expression of the HLA determinant on the human breast carcinoma cell line MCF-7 by 2–5-fold, whereas IFN-αD and -αJ had little if any effect, although they did bind to the IFN receptor. IFN-αC, -αF, -αI, and -αK had an intermediate effect. The ability of the IFNs to inhibit the proliferation of MCF-7 cells appeared to vary independently of their ability to augment HLA expression (Greiner *et al.*, 1986).

Human thymocytes cultured *in vitro* for 2 days express a more mature phenotype (low HTA 1, high T3 and HLA-A,B,C) than uncultured thymocytes (Diaz-Espada *et al.*, 1986). Culturing in the presence of IFN-α increases markedly the number of HLA-positive cells and the total amount of HLA expressed by the cultured cells. The cortical, immature thymocyte is the target cell for IFN action (Diaz-Espada *et al.*, 1986). IFN treatment of thymocytes diminishes their phytohaemagglutinin response, but not their IL-2 response. IFN appears to favour a pathway of intrathymic differentiation phenotypically characterized by a high content of class I HLA antigens (Diaz-Espada *et al.*, 1986).

Using a monoclonal antibody (W6/32) to HLA-A,B,C, and another monoclonal antibody (YT76) which recognizes a subset of HLA strongly induced by IFN-α, spontaneous mutants with altered HLA-A,B,C responses to IFN-α have been isolated from the human thymus leukaemia cell line Molt 4 with the aid of a fluorescence-activated cell sorter (Burrone *et al.*, 1985). With monoclonal antibody W6/32, mutant clones with low or high HLA responses to IFN-α were obtained after several cycles of selection. With YT76, stable clones were obtained in which a marked increase in the level of HLA-A,B,C expression after IFN-α treatment could be mostly accounted for by an increase in the expression of a subset of HLA molecules, detected by the monoclonal antibody YT76, including HLA-B molecules (Burrone *et al.*, 1985).

IFN-α, -β, and -γ all induce the expression of class I but not class II HLA antigens on the surface of K562 cells, a line of human leukaemic cells (Sutherland *et al.*, 1985; Garson *et al.*, 1985). These cells may be regarded as pluripotent haematopoietic progenitors because they have the capacity to differentiate along erythroid, macrophage and megakaryocytic lineages. K562 cells are usually considered as both class I and class II HLA-negative cells (Sutherland *et al.*, 1985; Garson *et al.*, 1985). In this system, IFNs either had no clear differentiating capacity as defined by the expression of various haematopoietic markers (Garson *et al.*, 1985) or had some differentiating capacity (Sutherland *et al.*, 1986). As class II HLA antigen expression could also not be induced by chemical differentiation induction (Sutherland *et al.*, 1985; Garson *et al.*, 1985), it appears that these cells may be defective with respect to the class II HLA genes, as is the case for β_2-microglobulin in Daudi cells.

Human small-cell lung cancer lines and fresh tumour samples are markedly deficient in expression of class I HLA-A,B,C antigens and β_2-microglobulin, whereas lung cancers of other types, including adenocarcinoma, epidermoid carcinoma, and large-cell carcinoma are not (Doyle *et al.*, 1985). The great majority of the small-cell lung cancer lines show markedly decreased amounts of HLA and β_2-microglobulin mRNA. IFN-α increased the expression of HLA-A,B,C and β_2-microglobulin surface antigens in the small-cell lung tumour lines. These findings raise the possibility that an E1a-like product (see Section II-C) may be present in this type of tumour cell and be responsible for the decreased expression of histocompatibility antigens (Doyle *et al.*, 1985).

Besides IFNs, TNF also increases the expression of class I HLA mRNA (Collins *et al.*, 1986); however, as was discussed above, this effect of TNF is mediated via induction of the synthesis of IFN-β_2 (May *et al.*, 1986). Modulation of the expression of the HLA genes could regulate the recognition of foreign antigens by cytotoxic T lymphocytes. The products of the class I genes are required for the presentation not only of virus-infected cells but also of tumour cells to the immune system (Zinkernagel and Doherty, 1979).

In human T98G neuroblastoma cells treated with IFN-α, seven different mRNAs are induced, which accumulate for about a day in the continued presence of IFN, but whose accumulation ceases when IFN is removed (Friedman *et al.*, 1984). The concentration of IFN-α required for half-maximal induction of metallothionein-II gene transcription is 30 times greater than that required for similar induction of HLA genes. A homologous sequence of $\sim$30 base pairs is present upstream of two class I HLA genes, one class II HLA gene and the metallothionein-II gene (Friedman and Stark, 1985). This sequence may be involved in the regulation of transcription of the IFN-induced genes.

Recently, evidence has been obtained that the target sequence required for enhancement of the accumulation of class I transcripts by IFN in mouse cells resides, at least in part, within the same 350-base pair segment which contains the transcriptional enhancer (Vogel *et al.*, 1986). This is in agreement with evidence showing that, in a DNA plasmid construct in which the 5′ flanking segment of an IFN-inducible murine gene (gene 202) was linked to the chloramphenicol acetyltransferase gene (Samanta *et al.*, 1986), the gene segment rendering the expression of the chloramphenicol acetyltransferase gene inducible by IFN had enhancer-like characteristics (G. Gribaudo and P. Lengyel, cited in Lengyel, 1986). This segment could activate heterologous promoters, and it was active in both the direct and the inverted orientation and in either upstream or downstream locations from the promoter that was activated.

In parallel with the induction of mRNA coding for HLA-A,B,C antigens

(Fellous *et al.*, 1982a), IFN-α and -β also markedly increase the amount of tubulin mRNA in human Ramos lymphoblastoid cells (Fellous *et al.*, 1982b). As with HLA-A,B,C mRNAs, the extent of induction of translatable tubulin mRNA is less pronounced than that of induction of tubulin mRNA sequences, detected by hybridization with the tubulin cDNA probe. IFN increases the level of α-tubulin mRNA more than β-tubulin mRNA, which suggests that the genes for the two tubulins may be regulated independently (Cleveland *et al.*, 1980, 1981; Fellous *et al.*, 1982b).

2 *Class II HLA*

IFN-γ induces HLA-DR (λ243) antigen biosynthesis and expression in normal cultured human keratinocytes within 1–2 days, with maximum expression observed after 4–8 days (Basham *et al.*, 1985). Little expression of another class II antigen, i.e. HLA-DC (Leu^{10}) was detected although Fc receptors for the IgG_1 isotype were increased. IFN-α or -β, interleukin 2, concanavalin A and phytohaemagglutinin failed to induce HLA-DR antigen expression in keratinocytes (Basham *et al.*, 1985; Auböck *et al.*, 1985). Incubation for a minimum of 3 hours with IFN-γ, followed by 72 hours in IFN-γ-free medium was sufficient to induce HLA-DR antigen expression (Auböck *et al.*, 1985). Melanocytes react identically to keratinocytes (Auböck *et al.*, 1985). Induction of HLA-DR may serve to expand the number of antigen-presenting cells in the skin preparatory to an immune response or for targetting of cells for cytolysis.

IFN-γ, but not IFN-α, induces HLA-DR antigen expression on those dendritic epidermal cells on which such antigens are normally not detected (Berman *et al.*, 1985). IFN-γ effectively induces HLA-DR on both neonatal and adult Langerhans cells. Such induction is inhibited by prostaglandin E2 and is mimicked by fatty acid cyclooxygenase inhibitors known to reduce prostaglandin E2 production (Berman *et al.*, 1985). The ability of Langerhans cells to function as accessory/stimulatory cells in initiating the immune response is, like that of macrophages, dependent on the expression of class II HLA antigens. Thus, IFN-γ may play a role in regulating skin-associated immune responses through enhanced expression of HLA-DR on Langerhans cells.

IFN-γ induces the expression of class II HLA antigens HLA-DR, HLA-DP, and HLA-DQ on cultured human vascular endothelial cells and the adhesion of lymphocytes to the endothelial cells, whereas IFN-α does not (Masuyama *et al.*, 1986). The lymphocyte adhesion is inhibited by monoclonal anti-HLA-DR antibody, but not by antibodies to HLA-DP, HLA-DQ, or HLA-A,B,C. The majority of lymphocytes that adhere to endothelial cells expressing class II HLA antigens are Leu-3+ T cells, and anti-Leu-3a, but not anti-Leu-2a, antibody inhibits their adhesion. These results indicate that interaction of the Leu-3(T4) receptor of T cells with the IFN-γ induced DR antigens on the endothelial cell surface plays a key role in the selective adhesion of Leu-3+ T cells to the endothelial cells (Masuyama *et al.*, 1986).

IFN-α and -β, but not IFN-γ, inhibit the proliferative response of human peripheral blood leukocytes to phytohaemagglutinin while inducing 2′,5′A synthetase activity in the cells (Billard *et al.*, 1986). However, all three IFNs enhance natural killer cell cytotoxicity and the expression of HLA-DR antigens.

In human breast cancer cell lines, HLA-DR expression is exclusively inducible by human IFN-γ (Gastl *et al.*, 1985). Induction of HLA-DR by IFN-γ does not correlate with antiproliferative activity, nor does it depend on proliferation; it does depend on RNA and protein synthesis and the continued presence of IFN-γ. IFN-γ and IFN-α_2 show differences in their antiproliferative action in terms of dose dependence and the cell spectrum. Combinations of IFN-γ and -α are more effective in inhibiting cell proliferation than either agent alone.

IFN-γ, but not IFN-α or -β, induces class II HLA antigen expression in human melanoma, osteogenic sarcoma, colorectal carcinoma, and glioma cell lines that are not constitutive producers of these antigens (Carrell *et al.*, 1985; Shaw *et al.*, 1985). However, in a cell line (SW480), which constitutively expressed low levels of HLA-DR, both IFN-γ and -β enhanced the expression of class II antigens (Shaw *et al.*, 1985). Moreover, IFN-γ, -α and -β all enhanced the synthesis of heavy chain and light chain (β_2-microglobulin) components and the cell surface expression of class I HLA antigens on a variety of tumour cell lines, although IFN-γ showed greatest activity (Shaw *et al.*, 1985; Carrel *et al.*, 1985). Enhancement of class I membrane expression preceded the induction of class II expression and peaked earlier in systems where both responses occurred (Shaw *et al.*, 1985; Carrel *et al.*, 1985).

Comparative studies of the effects of IFNs on three subsets of class II HLA molecules, i.e., DR, BR, and DQ, in a melanoma and a lymphoblastoid cell line and peripheral blood mononuclear cells of human origin showed that IFN-γ markedly increases class II HLA molecules, that IFN-β has a smaller enhancing effect, and that IFN-α is without effect or has only a slight effect as measured by cellular expression or shedding of the class II HLA molecules (Capobianchi *et al.*, 1985). Both IFN-γ and -β have a much greater effect on DQ than on either DR or BR expression.

3 2′,5′ oligoadenylate synthetase

The investigation of the 2′,5′ oligoadenylate synthetase system has received new impetus from the demonstration that different mRNAs exist (St Laurent *et al.*, 1983), which are translated into different isoenzymes (Benech *et al.*, 1985a). Some but not all of the different mRNAs arise through splicing of the same primary transcript in different ways (Benech *et al.*, 1985a; Chebath *et al.*, 1987). Some of the 2′,5′A isoenzymes are primarily nuclear whereas others are cytoplasmic (St Laurent *et al.*, 1983; Chebath *et al.*, 1986, 1987). Differences have been demonstrated in the concentration of dsRNA required for their activation (Ilson *et al.*, 1986).

Several studies have given results consistent with the notion that 2′,5′A synthetase may play a role in relation to cell cycle activity (reviewed in Tamm *et al.*, 1987). At the same time, attempts to link 2′,5′A synthetase levels, without distinguishing among the isoenzymes, to the inhibition of cell proliferation by IFN, have had inconclusive results, in that IFN increases 2′,5′A synthetase levels not only in IFN-sensitive, but also in IFN-resistant, Daudi lymphoblastoid cells. This has led to the tentative conclusion that induction of 2′,5′A synthetase by IFN either does not play a role in the antiproliferative effects of IFN in some cell lines or that it is not, alone, sufficient to account for the effects (Vandenbussche *et al.*, 1981; Verhaegen-Lewalle *et al.*, 1980). Recent evidence indicates that the patterns of IFN-induced protein synthesis are both quantitatively and qualitatively different in sensitive versus resistant Daudi cells (Dron *et al.*, 1985).

New and relevant information concerning the relationship of the 2′,5′A system to the cell cycle has come from studies of tertiary cultures of mouse embryo fibroblasts synchronized by controlling cultural conditions (Mallucci *et al.*, 1983; Wells and Mallucci, 1985; Mallucci *et al.*, 1985, 1986). After initial passages under appropriate conditions, the tertiary cells were seeded at a density such that a confluent monolayer was obtained after one division cycle. Such cells enter S phase with a high degree of synchrony at about 12 hours after seeding and complete the replication cycle at 28–30 hours. Addition of IFN to the synchronized nonconfluent cells results in an extension of the G_1 and G_2 phases of the cell cycle as determined by fluorimetric quantitation of cellular DNA (Mallucci *et al.*, 1983). The duration of the S phase is not extended regardless of whether IFN is added in early G_1 or at the beginning of S. However, IFN treatment does decrease thymidine uptake and delays the S phase-associated increase in thymidine kinase activity.

A 1.7 kb 2′,5′A synthetase RNA is present at low levels in confluent G_0 phase cells and its abundance does not change appreciably through the cell cycle (Mallucci *et al.*, 1986) as determined by hybridization with human 2′,5′A synthetase cDNAs (Merlin *et al.*, 1983; Benech *et al.*, 1985a). In contrast, a 4 kb transcript and a >5 kb transcript are present only during S and early G_2 phases. The 4 kb transcript may be a processing product of the

>5 kb RNA, and the active mRNA for 2′,5′A synthetase during S phase (Mallucci *et al.*, 1986). Consistent with these findings, cell-associated 2′,5′A synthetase activity is low in G_0 and G_1, but it increases markedly during S phase (Wells and Mallucci, 1985). In spite of the 10-fold increase in 2′,5′A synthetase level late in S phase, no phosphorylated 2′,5′A is detectable in the intact cells down to nM levels (Wells and Mallucci, 1985). Evidence of the presence of 2′,5′A cores has been obtained, but only at the limit of detection, and therefore is of uncertain significance. In S phase the level of 2′,5′A-dependent RNase is also increased, but less than that of 2′,5′A synthetase. In contrast, the activity of 2′,5′A phosphodiesterase is highest in quiescent G_0 cells. Cell culture supernatants show the presence of endogenously produced murine IFN, and the concentration of this IFN increases as the cell cycle progresses (Wells and Mallucci, 1985).

Exogenously added mouse IFN (prepared from BALB/c mouse cells infected with Newcastle disease virus) causes a marked increase in the cell cycle-independent 1.7 kb RNA species in cultures of mouse embryo fibroblasts (Mallucci *et al.*, 1986). Exogenous IFN strongly induces this RNA species also in mouse L cells (Mallucci *et al.*, 1985).

The 1.7 kb and 4 kb RNAs detected in tertiary mouse embryonic cells are similar to the 1.5 kb and 3.8 kb mRNAs whose levels increase in mouse Ehrlich ascites tumour (EAT) cells in response to IFN (St Laurent *et al.*, 1983). The 1.5 kb and 3.8 kb mRNAs of the EAT cells encode a nuclear 20–30 kD 2′,5′A synthetase and a cytoplasmic 85–100 kD 2′,5′A synthetase, respectively. The roles of these distinct 2′,5′A synthetase species are not known. The rapid disappearance of the 4 and >5 kb transcripts in the G_2 phase and the concurrent fall in the 2′,5′A synthetase level suggest that the functional scope of this enzyme is tightly controlled (Mallucci *et al.*, 1986).

In human cells, the 1.8 kb mRNA shares most of the sequence of a 1.6 kb mRNA, but contains an additional 3′ exon absent in the 1.6 kb mRNA, and the respective enzymes have different *C*-termini (Benech *et al.*, 1985a, b). It has been proposed that in human cells the 2′,5′A synthetase mRNAs of 1.6 kb and 1.8 kb are produced from a single 13.5 kb gene by the process of differential splicing between the seventh and an additional eighth exon of this gene (Benech *et al.*, 1985a, b). Also produced are several longer transcripts. The 1.6 and 1.8 kb mRNAs have been found in two human fibroblastic cell lines, but only the 1.8 kb RNA was detected in three lymphoblastoid B cell lines, and only the 1.6 mRNA in a histiocytic and an amniotic cell line (Benech *et al.*, 1985b). The sequences of the cDNA clones for the 1.6 kb and 1.8 kb mRNAs indicate that the 2′,5′A synthetase gene codes for two forms of the enzyme, of molecular weight 40–41 kD and 46 kD, which differ only by their *C*-terminal ends (Benech *et al.*, 1985a; Chebath *et al.*, 1986). The *C*-terminus in the product of the 1.6 kb mRNA is very hydrophobic, and could presumably bind to lipid membranes. In the 1.8 kb mRNA product this has been replaced by a longer acidic *C*-terminal sequence, which may allow interaction with ribosomes or basic proteins (Benech *et al.*, 1985a). A peptide common to the cDNAs for the 1.6 kb and 1.8 kb mRNAs has been synthesized and used to raise antibodies (Chebath *et al.*, 1986). These antibodies detect at least four different IFN-induced proteins in immunoblots of extracts of human cells. The mobilities in SDS-polyacrylamide gels correspond to 40, 46, 67 and 100 kD. Each of these proteins has 2′,5′A synthetase activity. The 67 kD 2′,5′A synthetase is ubiquitous, but the 100, 46 and 40 kD forms display a cell-specific expression. The four 2′,5′A synthetases differ in preferential intracellular localization (cell sap, ribosomes, nuclei, membranes), in dsRNA requirements, and in optimal conditions for activity. The same antibodies detect multiple forms of 2′,5′A synthetase in mouse cells (Chebath *et al.*, 1986, 1987).

A 30 kD and a 70 kD 2′,5′A synthetase have been described in a pool of cytoplasmic and ribosomal fractions of HeLa cells (Revel *et al.*, 1981). Another group of investigators has isolated a 20–30 kD enzyme from the HeLa cell nuclear fraction and an 80–100 kD enzyme from the cytoplasmic fraction (St Laurent *et al.*, 1983; Yang *et al.*, 1981). The smaller form corresponds in size to the proteins defined by cDNA sequencing (Benech *et al.*, 1985b). The identity of the larger of the two native enzyme forms remains to be determined. The 100–105 kD 2′,5′A synthetase from human cells has been purified to homogeneity, and the requirements for its activation have been characterized (Yang *et al.*, 1981; Wells *et al.*, 1984; Samanta *et al.*, 1986).

A comparison of the activation requirements of partially purified 33 kD and 110 kD 2′,5′A synthetases from HeLa cells has shown that the 33 kD enzyme is optimally activated only at concentrations of dsRNA 100–1000 times greater than those activating the 110 kD enzyme (Ilson *et al.*, 1986). Thus, it is not possible to assay accurately for both enzymes simultaneously under a single set of conditions. The assay conditions commonly used would favour the higher molecular weight species of 2′,5′A synthetase and might result in failure to detect the lower molecular weight species (Ilson *et al.*, 1986). Another difference between the two species is that poly(A:U) or poly(A:U:I) activate only the 100 kD enzyme (Ilson *et al.*, 1986). These differences would permit independent regulation of the lower and the higher molecular weight species of 2′,5′A synthetase.

In actively dividing NIH 3T3 clone 1 cells, the levels of 2′,5′A-dependent RNase are low (Krause *et al.*, 1985). They are induced independently by growth arrest and by IFN treatment. In confluent, growth-arrested cells the increase in 2′,5′A-dependent RNase is not prevented by antibody to IFN in the medium.

It is evident that a meaningful analysis of the role of 2′,5′A synthetases in cellular physiology and the action of IFNs can only be carried out when the multiplicity and the diverse properties of the enzymes are taken into account.

IV HOW CAN IFN EFFECTS BE COUNTERACTED?

IFNs are capable of antagonizing the cell growth-stimulating activity of a number of factors, including PDGF (Inglot *et al.*, 1980; Oleszak and Inglot, 1980; Einat *et al.*, 1985a; Lin *et al.*, 1985, 1986a), EGF (Lin *et al.*, 1983b), TNF (Sugarmen *et al.*, 1985; Vilček *et al.*, 1986), and insulin (Pfeffer *et al.*, 1986, 1987b), among others. IFNs can suppress the stimulation of thymidine incorporation by a combination of three growth factors (EGF, insulin and vasopressin) or by a combination of insulin and the tumour promoter TPA (Sreevalsan *et al.*, 1980). However, the inhibitory action of IFNs can be overcome by the use of combinations of several growth factors, or of relatively high growth factor/IFN concentration ratios. It also appears that some factors (such as PDGF and IL-1) may have greater ability than others to counteract IFN action.

IFN treatment was unable to affect the stimulation of thymidine incorporation by a combination of five growth factors in mouse 3T3 cells (EGF, insulin, vasopressin, colchicine, fibroblast growth factor) (Taylor-Papadimitriou *et al.*, 1981). Depending on concentrations of the agents and the system used, PDGF can be shown to inhibit or overcome IFN action (Oleszak and Inglot, 1980; Tamm *et al.*, unpublished). EGF has been reported to be able to overcome the inhibition of Madin-Darby bovine kidney cell growth by IFN-α_2 (Zoon *et al.*, 1986a). PDGF and IL-1 can override the IFN-β_2-mediated antiviral effect of IFN and also that of exogenously added IFN-β_1 in human FS-4 fibroblasts (Kohase *et al.*, 1987a). In line with the ability of growth factors to act as IFN antagonists, the antiproliferative effect of IFN-α/β on early murine bone marrow-derived erythroid precursors can be blocked by ouabain (Gallien-Lartigue *et al.*, 1985). Furthermore, the growth-inhibitory effect of IFN was more pronounced when the cells were cultured in the presence of suboptimal concentrations of erythropoietin.

Several viruses appear to possess a mechanism for counteracting the activation of the IFN-induced Pl/eIF-2α kinase. Mengovirus RNA can inhibit the dsRNA-dependent phosphorylation of P1 and eIF-2α polypeptides in reticulocyte lysates (Rosen *et al.*, 1981). A factor accumulates in vaccinia virus-infected cells that prevents activation of the P1/eIF-2α kinase (Paez and Esteban, 1984; Rice and Kerr, 1984; Whitaker-Dowling and Younger, 1983, 1984). Adenovirus-associated (VA) I RNA may also prevent activation of the kinase by dsRNA (Kitajewski *et al.*, 1986a). IFN does not inhibit the replication of wild-type virus, but the growth of a viral mutant that is unable to produce the small VAI RNA is inhibited by IFN in 293 cells, but not in KB cells (Kitajewski *et al.*, 1986b). The two small Epstein-Barr virus-encoded RNAs (EBER) are structurally similar to VA RNAs (Lerner *et al.*, 1981; Rosa *et al.*, 1981) and can partially substitute for VAI RNA in adenovirus-infected cells (Bhat and Thimmappaya 1983, 1985).

V WHAT ARE THE PHYSIOLOGICAL INDUCERS OF IFNs?

A Induction of IFNs by Cell Growth Factors and Proteins with Growth Factor Activity

In a study designed to obtain evidence of endogenous IFN as a counter-regulatory factor that might play a role in the mitogenic processes governed by EGF, evidence was obtained that EGF causes a three- to five-fold increase in 2′,5′A synthetase (Lin *et al.*, 1983b). This occurred early in the course of induction of S phase entry of quiescent human fibroblasts. Although EGF stimulation did not result in the secretion of detectable amounts of IFN, and although anti-IFN-β antibodies did not block the EGF-mediated increase in 2′,5′A synthetase, such antibodies did prolong the time course of EGF-stimulated DNA synthesis in human as well as in Syrian hamster embryo fibroblasts, and the effect of the anti-IFN-β antibodies could be reversed by the addition of IFN-β (Lin *et al.*, 1983b).

Tumour necrosis factor (TNF) exerts a mitogenic effect in confluent cultures of human diploid fibroblasts (Sugarman *et al.*, 1985; Vilček *et al.*, 1986). In such cultures TNF also has an inhibitory effect on encephalomyocarditis virus and herpes virus replication (Kohase *et al.*, 1986). Addition of neutralizing antibodies against human IFN-β completely blocks the antiviral effect of TNF and also enhances the mitogenic action of TNF (Kohase *et al.*, 1986). Thus, induction of IFN-β appears to be a negative feedback mechanism regulating TNF-stimulated cell proliferation. Of special interest is the finding that TNF specifically induces the expression of the human IFN-β_2 gene, and not that of the IFN-β_1 gene, as determined by blot hybridization analysis of cytoplasmic polyadenylated RNA (Kohase *et al.*, 1986).

It has recently been demonstrated that IL-1 specifically induces IFN-β_2 in human fibroblasts (Content *et al.*, 1985; Kohase *et al.*, 1987a, b, c). IL-1 can itself be induced by TNF (Bachwich *et al.*, 1986; Nawroth *et al.*, 1986; Dinarello *et al.*, 1986; Le *et al.*, 1987). These aspects and the observation that IFN-β_1 induces IFN-β_2 and that TNF-induced IFN-β_2 expression can be enhanced by IFN-β_1 (Kohase *et al.*, 1987a) will be discussed in Section VI, which deals with the network of cytokines and their actions.

PDGF and calf serum induce the expression of the IFN-β_2 gene (but not the β_1 gene) in confluent, quiescent human fibroblasts (Kohase *et al.*, 1987a). In contrast, exposure of such cells to EGF does not lead to increased expression of IFN-β_2 mRNA (Kohase *et al.*, 1987b). In mouse BALB/c 3T3 cells, PDGF has been reported to induce IFN-β_1 mRNA (Zullo *et al.*, 1985), but this observation remains to be substantiated.

Evidence has been obtained recently that suggests the involvement of protein kinase C activation in the induction of IFN-β_2 (Sehgal *et al.*, 1987b). The synthetic diacylglycerols, 1,2-dioctanoylglycerol (DiC_8) and 1-oleoyl-2-acetylglycerol (OAG) strongly enhance IFN-β_2 mRNA expression in human fibroblasts (FS-4 cells derived from foreskin). The increase in IFN-β_2 mRNA levels in response to DiC_8 can be blocked by 1-(5-isoquinolinesulphonyl)-2-methylpiperazine dihydrochloride (H7), an inhibitor of protein kinase C as well as of cyclic nucleotide-dependent protein kinases, but not by *N*[2-(methylamino)ethyl]-5-isoquinolinesulphonamide dihydrochloride (H8), a preferential inhibitor of cyclic AMP- or GMP-dependent protein kinases. DiC_8, in the same concentration range that causes the induction of IFN-β_2 mRNA (1–100 μg/ml), elicits an antiviral state in FS-4 cells against vesicular stomatitis virus. The antiviral activity of DiC_8 can be blocked by anti-IFN-β monoclonal or polyclonal antibodies included in the culture medium (Sehgal *et al.*, 1987b). TPA also induces IFN-β_2 in human lymphocytes (Hirano *et al.*, 1986). The exquisite responsiveness of the IFN-β_2 gene to activation of protein kinase C may explain why this gene is induced by several different growth stimulatory cytokines such as PDGF, TNF and IL-1.

As cells of the mononuclear phagocyte system mature and differentiate, they progressively lose their capacity to proliferate in response to the growth factor known as colony-stimulating factor 1 (CSF-1) or macrophage growth factor, even though more mature, differentiated macrophages continue to express receptors for CSF-1 (reviewed in Moore *et al.*, 1984). However, in the more differentiated cells, CSF-1 can induce various functional changes, including secretion of series E prostaglandins, IL-1, and IFN. These findings illustrate how one and the same factor can act either as a proliferative signal for precursor or immature cells, or as a signal for the expression of specific functions in more differentiated cells.

Recent evidence indicates that IFN plays at least two roles in the process involving CSF-1 stimulation of committed stem cells and mature mononuclear cells (Moore *et al.*, 1985). Prostaglandin E and IFN produced by mature cells in haematopoietic tissues when they are locally exposed to CSF-1 can suppress CSF-induced colony formation *in vitro* in a negative feedback manner. Murine IFN-α/β decreases the number of cell surface receptors for CSF-1 on murine peritoneal exudate macrophages and also inhibits the receptor-mediated endocytosis of CSF-1 in macrophages. Since the continuous presence of CSF-1 is required for the proliferation of macrophage stem cells, IFN may inhibit proliferation of these cells by down-modulating CSF-1 receptors and by inhibiting CSF-1 uptake (Chen, 1986). The endogeneous IFN produced by mature cells also enhances functional maturation of the monocyte progeny, and thus acts as a differentiation signal for immature cells of the same lineage that respond to the growth stimulus of CSF-1 (Moore *et al.*, 1985). Notably, when cultures are deprived of IFN during clonal expansion, the cells display severely depressed capacities to produce IL-1, to resist lytic herpes virus infection, and to phagocytize opsonized erythrocytes via Fc receptors.

In cultures of murine femoral marrow cells, evidence has been obtained that the IFN produced in response to CSF-1 in the more differentiated adherent cells (including macrophages and monocytes) inhibits the growth response of committed precursor cells to CSF-1 (Moore *et al.*, 1984). Production of IFN by the adherent cells was demonstrated by antiviral assays and neutralization of the endogenous IFN produced with antiserum directed against IFN-α and -β. The IFN produced was subsequently identified as murine IFN-β (Resnitzky *et al.*, 1986). The cell growth inhibitory action of the endogenous IFN was established both by [^{3}H]thymidine incorporation and by colony formation assays carried out in the absence or presence of anti-IFN antibodies.

Previously, series E prostaglandins produced by CSF-induced macrophages had been implicated in a negative regulatory role (Kurland *et al.*, 1978; Pelus *et al.*, 1979), and evidence was obtained that macrophages within the marrow can act as suppressors of the myelopoietic response (Spitzer *et al.*, 1981; Broxmeyer *et al.*, 1982). The relative contributions of series E prostaglandins and IFN to the regulation of CSF-induced macrophage proliferation remain to be determined (Moore *et al.*, 1984).

B Induction IFNs by Differentiation Factors and Other Physiological Agents

Mouse myeloid leukaemic M1 cells, induced to differentiate into phagocytic cells by incubation with conditioned medium from rat embryo cells, show an increase in 2′,5′A synthetase, which can be suppressed with anti-IFN antibody without affecting the phagocytic activity of the cells (Sokawa *et al.*, 1981). Since IFNs have been shown to stimulate phagocytosis (reviewed in Wang *et al.*, 1984), the significance of the lack of an anti-IFN antibody effect on the phagocytic activity of M1 cells induced to differentiate is complex. IFN activity is detectable in cell extracts, but not in the culture medium. Antibodies to IFN-β restore only a part of the cellular proliferative activity and c-*myc* exprssion in M1 myeloid cells induced to differentiate by lung-conditioned medium, suggesting that the differentiating cells produce additional growth inhibitors that may function together with the autocrine IFN in causing a complete growth arrest of cells (Resnitzky *et al.*, 1986).

2′,5′A synthetase also increases in Friend erythroleukaemia cells stimulated to differentiate by dimethyl sulphoxide (Friedman-Einat *et al.*, 1982; Kimchi *et al.*, 1983). The increase appears to be due to production of IFN-β. Differentiation is associated with a marked reduction in p53 synthesis as the cells become arrested in the G_0/G_1 phase. Similar findings have been obtained in human U937 cells which are derived from a histiocytic lymphoma and can be induced to differentiate by TPA towards macrophage-like cells (Kimchi *et al.*, 1983; Yarden *et al.*, 1984; Ferbus *et al.*, 1985). The increase in 2′,5′A synthetase in the U937 cells induced to differentiate precedes the expression of several of the differentiation markers (Ferbus *et al.*, 1985). Prevention of increased expression of the genes for 2′,5′A synthetase and class I HLA by antibodies to IFN-β does not affect the morphological differentiation of the cells. Induction of the class I HLA and 2′,5′A synthetase genes by endogenously produced IFN differs with respect to the dose–response sensitivity and the prolonged kinetics of mRNA accumulation from the response to exogenous IFN-β (Resnitzky *et al.*, 1986).

VI WHERE DO IFNs FIT IN AMONG CYTOKINES?

Cytokines represent a class of inducible proteins that play a role in the host response to infectious agents and in other situations. Numerous cytokines exist and are produced in a wide variety of cell types, including epithelial cells, fibroblasts, tumour cells, lymphocytes (lymphokines), and macrophages (monokines). One cell may produce several different cytokines. IFN-α, -β and -γ species, along with TNF, LT, IL-1α and IL-1β, are among the well-characterized cytokines. As cytokines regulate the production of one another, it can be difficult to establish the nature of the primary or direct action of a given cytokine.

IFNs appear to play several distinct roles within the complex network of cytokines and their actions. The findings summarized in Section V-A clearly show that IFN-β_2 produced in cells in response to growth factor action can exert negative feedback control over cell proliferation. This remarkable autocrine mechanism, serving to restrict the proliferative response of cells to cytokines with growth-stimulating activity, has thus far been firmly associated only with the novel human IFN-β_2 species.

A second demonstrated function of endogenously produced IFN is to mediate the effect of other cytokines on cellular properties. While the facts are clear, as exemplified by the role of IFN-β_2 in mediating the enhancement by TNF of class I HLA gene expression, the evolutionary origins and the relative physiological significance of mediation by IFN of the effects of other cytokines are not. Did IFN-β_2 evolve relatively recently as a gene with a function that enables the cell to regulate its proliferation more precisely, with the mediating function being a carry-over from earlier evolutionary times, when IFNs became endowed with the capability to increase class I HLA gene expression, and exert other effects on cells?

As other IFNs are capable of inhibiting cell proliferation when exogenously added to cells, the special position of the β_2-IFN gene with respect to cell growth regulation would appear to relate most importantly to factors that control the inducibility of this gene. However, the distinctive structural features appear to endow β_2-IFN with a number of special regulatory functions.

What is clear is that some of the growth factors that induce IFN-β_2, i.e., IL-1 and PDGF, are capable of counteracting some of the effects of the induced IFN-β_2 that are not directly related to regulation of cell growth. IL-1 and PDGF both induce IFN-β_2 mRNA without the concomitant development of an antiviral state in human diploid fibroblasts (Kohase *et al.*, 1987a), although in human osteosarcoma MG63 cells, IL-1 does induce an antiviral state mediated via IFN-β_2 (Content *et al.*, 1985; Kohase *et al.*, 1987c). TNF induces IL-1 expression in macrophages, endothelial cells and human fibroblasts (Bachwich *et al.*, 1986; Nawroth *et al.*, 1986; Dinarello *et al.*, 1986; Le *et al.*, 1987).

It is noteworthy that the expression of the antiviral action of TNF can be enhanced by prior exposure of human fibroblasts to trace amounts of IFN-β_1 (Kohase *et al.*, 1987a). Furthermore, at a higher concentration, IFN-β_1 can directly increase the expression of IFN-β_2 (Kohase *et al.*, 1987a). Interactions have also been observed among other IFNs.

The constitutive expression of IFN-β_2 in human monocytes (Sanceau *et al.*, 1986) and in normal human spleen (Tovey, 1986) suggests that this molecule may play a role in the regulation of macrophage function. The role of IFN-β_2 as the B-cell differentiation factor was discussed in Section II-B.

VII HOW IS THE EXPRESSION OF IFN GENES REGULATED?

The human IFN-β_1 gene contains regulatory sequences within its 5′-flanking region that mediate virus- or poly(I)·poly(C)-induced activation of mRNA transcription (Fujita *et al.*, 1985; Goodbourn *et al.*, 1985). Goodbourn *et al.* (1985) identified a sequence with the characteristics of an inducible enhancer element in the region between −37 and −77 from the mRNA cap site. On the other hand, Fujita *et al.* (1985) localized the inducible regulatory element in the IFN-β_1 gene to a region between -78 and -117 from the mRNA cap site. A regulatory element similar to the one described by Fujita *et al.* (1985) is present between -109 and -64 in the 5′-flanking region of the IFN-α_1 gene (Ryals *et al.*, 1985). All three laboratories report that the regulatory elements delineated by them confer poly(I)·poly(C) or virus inducibility to a heterologous promoter when used in their particular expression vector systems. Nevertheless, there is no satisfactory explanation, as yet, for the different results obtained by Fujita *et al.* (1985) and Goodbourn *et al.* (1985) in defining the regulatory region of the IFN-β_1 gene.

Maniatis and colleagues have continued their experiments in characterizing the -37 to -77 element in the IFN-β_1 gene in detail as it behaves in their bovine papilloma virus/β-globin expression vector (Goodbourn *et al.*, 1986; Zinn and Maniatis, 1986). Within this element there is present a minimal regulatory region of 14 base pairs. The 5′-flanking regions of both the IFN-α and -β genes contain multiple copies of sequences closely related to the 14-base pair element. The enhancer element is under negative control as deletion of sequences from the 3′ end of the enhancer (-55 to -36) results in a marked increase in the basal level of IFN-β mRNA and a decrease in the induction ratio (Goodbourn *et al.*, 1986). The remaining 5′ region of the enhancer (-77 to -55) can act as a constitutive transcription element. It appears that depression of the constitutive transcription element plays a key role in the control of human IFN-β gene expression. Further evidence in support of this conclusion has come from the use of a DNase 1 genomic footprinting procedure to detect interactions between cellular factors and the regulatory sequences in MG63 osteosarcoma cells (Zinn and Maniatis, 1986). Prior to induction of MG63 cells with poly(I)·poly(C), two factors can be detected which are bound, respectively, to one region located between -94 and -167 from the mRNA cap site, and to another region located between -68 and -38. These factors disassociate after induction, and another factor binds to a region located between -77 and -64. Taken together, the results suggest that the factors that bind prior to induction are repressor molecules, whereas the factor that binds after induction is a transcription factor (Zinn and Maniatis, 1986). It is not clear to what extent these data obtained in MG63 cells can be extrapolated to normal diploid fibroblasts and how these data can be reconciled with those of Fujita *et al.* (1985).

Priming of human fibroblasts with homologous IFN (100 U/ml) prior to induction with poly(I)·poly(C) increases the levels of induced IFN-β_1 mRNA 5–10-fold; this results mainly from an increased transcription rate of the IFN-β_1 gene (Nir *et al.*, 1985). Earlier studies showed that priming of IFN-β_1 mRNA accumulation is dependent on protein synthesis (Raj and Pitha, 1983). A poly(I)·poly(C)-inducible gene has been identified next to the 3′ end of the IFN-β_1 gene, which is highly activated in cells primed with IFN, while the expression of another poly(I)·poly(C)-inducible gene located on a different chromosome is only slightly affected by such priming (Nir *et al.*, 1985). It thus appears that priming only acts on certain genes and does not lead to a general potentiation of the expression of genes inducible by poly(I)·poly(C). Priming also leads to elevated cytoplasmic steady-state levels of two additional RNA species that initiate at the major IFN-β_1 initiation site and extend beyond the polyadenylation site for the 0·9 kb IFN-β_1 mRNA (Nir *et al.*, 1985).

The 5′-flanking and promoter regions of the human IFN-β_2 gene contain contiguous nucleotide-sequence elements that have distinctive similarities with the serum-responsive enhancer element in the human c-*fos* gene (from −109 to −124), the Spl transcription factor binding GC-box sequence (from −123 to −98), and the poly(I)·poly(C) and virus-inducible enhancer element in the human IFN-β_1 gene (from −97 to −39) (Walther *et al.*, 1987). This "complex" regulatory region is consistent with the inference, drawn from cycloheximide experiments, that IL-1 and TNF increase IFN-β_2 gene transcription in human fibroblasts by different mechanisms (Walther *et al.*, 1987). The enhancing effect of IL-1 on IFN-β_2 transcription is decreased by cycloheximide, whereas that of TNF is not. This suggests that a newly synthesized protein mediates most of the increase in IFN-β_2 gene transcription in response to IL-1, but that the response to TNF is not mediated via a newly synthesized protein. Furthermore, IFN-β_2 gene transcription is sustained at a high level for at least 14 hours in IL-1-treated fibroblasts, whereas the increase is transient following TNF addition and declines by 6 hours.

1,2-Dioctanoylglycerol and 1-oleoyl-2-acetyl-glycerol induce IFN-β_2 gene transcription within 5 minutes in human fibroblasts (Sehgal *et al.*, 1987b). The rate of IFN-β_2 transcription is maximal by 30 minutes after addition of these diacylglycerols to the cells. This experimental system is likely to prove valuable in delineating the biochemical basis of rapid signal transduction from the extracellular environment to a particular well-characterized gene.

VIII IFNs IN THE WHOLE ORGANISM

A Exogenously Induced or Administered IFNs

The ability of cells of a given type, derived from different individuals, to produce a particular IFN upon induction of the cells is a quantitatively graded character (Moehring *et al.*, 1971; Havel and Vilček, 1972). This is consistent with the view that the production of IFN is a polygenic, multifactorial trait. Some of the genes involved may well have several alleles, which would give rise to genetic polymorphism. However, the wide range of variation observed probably cannot be explained on the basis of multiple allelism alone.

Cells, both normal and transformed, vary widely in their sensitivity to IFNs. Variation among normal cells has been documented in several systems. IFN-β inhibition of erythropoietin-dependent colony formation by committed erythroid cells depends markedly on the genotype of the murine cell genome (Gallien-Lartigue *et al.*, 1980). The degree of IFN inhibition of growth-factor-dependent colony formation by bone marrow cells from normal human donors forms a continuum from none to marked inhibition (Bradley and Ruscetti, 1981). Human fibroblast lines from different donors show considerable differences in their sensitivity to the cell growth-inhibitory effect of IFN-β, while cells of a given fibroblast line do not vary significantly with the population doubling level of the culture line (Tamm *et al.*, 1984b). As the IFN sensitivity trait is clearly multifactorial and its inheritance is therefore polygenic, it would be expected that the frequency distribution of IFN sensitivity could be represented by the normal curve. Whether this is the case has not been determined. Nor is it known what role the differences in IFN sensitivity of tumour-bearing individuals play in the findings that IFN inhibition of colony formation by tumour cells of a given type (e.g. melanoma, ovarian carcinoma, or leukaemia), but obtained from different individuals, shows marked quantitative differences distributed over a wide range. There is evidence, however, that determination of IFN sensitivity of tumour cells from individual patients is useful for the identification of IFN responders in the clinic (Strayer *et al.*, 1984).

A start has been made in understanding the biochemical mechanisms underlying differences in IFN sensitivity and in utilizing such information in the selection of patients for IFN treatment of neoplastic diseases. It has been established that, in general, those patients with chronic myelogenous leukaemia who respond to IFN-α treatment show substantial induction of 2′,5′A synthetase in peripheral blood cells whereas nonresponders do not (Rosenblum *et al.*, 1986). However, some responders to IFN therapy showed no induction of 2′,5′A synthetase activity. No significant differences were found in the binding of IFN to cells from patients who showed a response to therapy as compared to those who did not respond and IFN receptor down-regulation following IFN administration occurred both in responders and nonresponders (Rosenblum *et al.*, 1986). Although IFN-α inhibits the growth, in culture, of colonies of granulocytes and monocytes from either normal donors or patients with chronic myelogenous leukaemia (Verma *et al.*, 1979; Neumann and Fauser, 1982; Oladipupo-Williams *et al.*, 1981), administration of IFN to responsive patients with Ph-chromosome-positive chronic myelogenous leakaemia appears to be associated with a selective cytoreductive effect on the Ph cells and haematologic remission (Talpaz *et al.*, 1983, 1986). In the Ph cells, the c-*abl* gene is translocated from chromosome 9 to chromosome 22 (Bartram *et al.*, 1983), where it codes for an abnormal message (Shtivelman *et al.*, 1985) and a novel protein with tyrosine kinase activity (Konopka *et al.*, 1984; Kloetzer *et al.*, 1985). It has been suggested, based on the ability of IFNs to suppress oncogene expression in other systems (Lin *et al.*, 1983a; Samid *et al.*, 1984; Jonak and Knight, 1984), that IFN treatment may suppress c-*abl* expression in chronic myelogenous leukaemia (Talpaz *et al.*, 1986).

IFN-α treatment of hairy cell leukaemia reduces the number of leukaemic cells and restores the levels of granulocytes, macrophages, platelets and haemoglobin (Quesada *et al.*, 1984; Jacobs *et al.*, 1985; Aderka *et al.*, 1985). IFN-γ is ineffective in the treatment of hairy cell leukaemia. Patients with this disease have circulating haematopoietic stem cells which give rise to mixed lymphomyeloid colonies *in vitro* (Revel and Michalevicz, 1986). IFN-αC decreases the number of lymphoid cells and increases the number of myeloid and monocytic cells without affecting the number of colonies or their size. IFN-β_1 has similar effects, whereas IFN-γ does not show such effects. It is possible that IFN-α and -β relieve a block in the differentiation of the haematopoietic stem cells towards the non-lymphoid lineages, thereby decreasing lymphogenesis.

Numerous attempts are now under way to increase desirable cell growth-inhibitory effects by combining IFN with other agents (reviewed in Hubbell, 1986). Mismatched dsRNA ($r(I)_n.r(C_{12}U)_n$), termed Ampligen) is rapidly cleared from blood and lacks the significant toxicity associated with dsRNA ($rI_n.rC_n$) or IFN administration to humans or animals (Carter *et al.*, 1985). Comparisons of the patterns of tumour cell sensitivity to IFNs and to mismatched dsRNA suggest that the dsRNA may have a mechanism of action apart from IFN induction. Not only are the sensitivities of cells to IFN and dsRNA often different (Lin *et al.*, 1982; Hubbel *et al.*, 1984), but, when combined, these agents frequently have a synergistic effect (Hubbell *et al.*, 1985, Hubbell, 1986). For example, various IFN preparations and mismatched dsRNA give a synergistic antiproliferative effect in the following human tumour cell lines: the RT4 bladder carcinoma line, which is IFN-sensitive and dsRNA-resistant; the lung carcinoma line A2182, which is IFN-resistant and dsRNA-sensitive; and the fibrosarcoma line HT1080C14, which shows some sensitivity to both IFN and mismatched dsRNA (Hubbell *et al.*, 1984; Hubbell, 1986). Mismatched dsRNA is much more effective than human IFN-α in increasing the survival of nude mice bearing human renal cell carcinoma xenographs (Carter *et al.*, 1985).

B Role of Endogenous IFNs

IFNs appear to be produced constitutively *in vivo* (Lebon *et al.*, 1981, 1982; Bocci *et al.*, 1984), and may play a role in host defence against viral infection and neoplasia, as well as in the physiological regulation of cell proliferation (Belardelli *et al.*, 1984; Gresser *et al.*, 1983; Yaar *et al.*, 1986). IFN-α has been detected in the amniotic fluid (Lebon *et al.*, 1981), and IFNs with the properties of either IFN-γ or an acid-labile IFN-α or a mixture have been found in the lymph of rabbits (Bocci *et al.*, 1984).

The transplantability of a variety of murine tumours in immunocompetent 5–8-week-old mice can be enhanced by injection of the mice with antibody to IFN-α/β, as indicated by an increase in the percentage of tumour-bearing mice and a decrease in survival time (Gresser *et al.*, 1983). The enhancement is most marked when the tumour cells used are of low tumorigenicity, and, as found out with Friend erythroleukaemia cells, when antibody is administered at the time of tumour cell injection. In some tumour systems, anti-IFN globulin has no effect (Gresser *et al.*, 1983). No biologically active IFN was detectable in peritoneal washings, splenic extracts or sera of mice before or after tumour cell inoculation. However, injection of several-week-old mice with antibody to IFN-α/β does decrease the basal level of 2′,5′A synthetase in resting peritoneal macrophages (Gresser *et al.*, 1985).

Vesicular stomatitis and encephalomyocarditis viruses are able to replicate only in a small fraction of freshly explanted peritoneal macrophages from 4–6-week-old mice (Belardelli *et al.*, 1984). However, these viruses can infect most of the macrophages from mice which have been injected several days earlier with anti-IFN-α/β globulin. In macrophages from such mice, high titres of virus are produced. Anti-IFN globulin also renders peritoneal macrophages susceptible to infection by vesicular stomatitis virus when infection is carred out *in vivo*.

There is an inverse correlation between the level of 2′,5′A synthetase in peritoneal macrophages and the susceptibility of the cells to infection with vesicular stomatitis virus (Gresser *et al.*, 1985). Macrophages from 1- and 2-week-old mice have low levels of 2′,5′A synthetase and are susceptible to infection with vesicular stomatitis virus, whereas cells from mice 3 weeks old or older have a markedly higher level of 2′,5′A synthetase and are no longer susceptible to the virus. mRNA hybridizing with the mouse IFN-α_2 gene DNA can be detected as a prominent species in the spleens of pathogen-free 4–6-week-old mice in the absence of induction (Tovey and Gresser, 1985). Some IFN-α_2 mRNA can also be detected in extracts of kidney, brain, liver, thymus and lung, but not in extracts of peritoneal cells or pancreas. No IFN-β_1 mRNA could be detected. The expression of IFN-β_2 in murine peritoneal macrophages remains to be measured.

IFN-α mRNA is detectable in spleens of accident victims and in peripheral blood leukocytes from normal adult donors (Tovey and Gresser, 1985). It forms a single distinct band of approximately 1.2 kb and hybridizes to human αC DNA. This RNA co-migrates with mature 1.2 kb IFN-α mRNA isolated from Newcastle disease virus-induced human peripheral blood leukocytes. No IFN-β_1 mRNA could be detected in human spleen cells or peripheral blood leukocytes without induction (Tovey and Gresser, 1985). However, IFN-β_2 mRNA is present constitutively at high levels (Tovey, 1986).

Although the normal epidermis renews itself continually, the majority of the cells in the germinative basal layer do not cycle unless stimulated (Grove *et al.*, 1976). These cells may be blocked in G_1, G_2 or G_0 phase. The basal layer of the epidermis and cultured keratinocyte colonies contain an IFN-like protein that reacts with polyclonal antibodies to recombinant human IFN-α (Yaar *et al.*, 1986). Extracts of cultured keratinocytes show antiviral activity and contain a 40 kD protein which is recognized by antibodies to IFN-α. Such antibodies recognize two bands (20 and 40 kD) in recombinant human IFN-α preparations (Yaar *et al.*, 1986). It has been suggested that the IFN-like protein serves as a growth regulator in the epidermis (Yaar *et al.*, 1986).

IFN-α species, both acid-stable and acid-labile, are found in sera from patients with polyclonal activation of B cells as a constitutive part of the disease. Systematic examination of a large number of human lymphoblastoid cell lines revealed that spontaneous production of IFN is common, as it could be detected in more than 50% of randomly procured lines (Pickering *et al.*, 1980). In many of the positive cultures, the levels of spontaneously produced IFN were higher than those obtainable in virus-induced lymphoblastoid cells. Lymphoblastoid cells produced IFN spontaneously only when growing exponentially. All the spontaneously produced IFNs were characterized as IFN-α species (Pickering *et al.*, 1980).

B cell lines established from patients with adult T-cell leukaemia, infected with human T cell leukaemia/lymphoma virus 1 (HTLV-1) or Epstein-Barr virus (EBV) or both, have been examined for the spontaneous production of IFN (Boumpas *et al.*, 1985). Among three B cell lines containing integrated HTLV-1 proviral sequences and infected with EBV, one (CF) produced and secreted acid-stable IFN-α, whereas two (HS and MJB) released acid-labile IFN-α. In contrast, HTLV-I-infected T cell lines did not produce IFN. Some EBV-infected B cell lines produce acid-labile IFN, but others do not. These observations suggest that polyclonal B cell activation may play a role in the production of IFN-α in these diseases (Boumpas *et al.*, 1985).

IX GENERAL DISCUSSION AND CONCLUSIONS

In the preceding sections we considered recent evidence with a view to arriving at insights as to how IFN-α and -β species operate as cellular regulatory molecules. The hypotheses or models that appear justified by current evidence should in each case be viewed as probably applicable to some or even an array of cell systems, but in all likelihood not to all possible systems. There is overwhelming evidence that the organisms and its tissues use multiple pathways for mediating and modulating the expression of its innate programmes as well as in responding to signals from the environment. It may be said that this is a requirement of homeostatic fine tuning.

A Pathways for Endogenous Induction of IFNs

The diacylglycerol-protein kinase C signal transduction pathway is one of the pathways that mediates the endogenous induction of IFNs in response to other cytokines, including growth factors. PDGF, which is known to stimulate inositol phospholipid turnover, induces IFN-β_2 in quiescent human diploid fibroblasts (Kohase *et al.*, 1987a), as do synthetic diacylglycerols (1,2-dioctanoylglycerol and 1-oleoyl-2-acetylglycerol) (Sehgal *et al.*, 1987b). There is indirect evidence that the effects of diacylglycerols are mediated via the activation of protein kinase C, and that protein kinase C activity is also involved in mediating the low-level constitutive expression of IFN-β_2 in these cells. TPA, which also activates protein kinase C, induces IFN-β_2 expression in human lymphocytes (Hirano *et al.*, 1986).

These findings point to the possibility that the IFN-β_2 gene could be induced by a variety of cytokines that may activate the diacylglycerol-protein kinase C pathway in cells. If agents such as TNF and IL-1, which, like PDGF, induce IFN-β_2 in quiescent human fibroblasts (Kohase *et al.*, 1987a), activate the diacylglycerol-protein kinase C pathway, this would provide a basis for explaining how diverse cytokines are able to activate IFN-β_2 gene transcription in a particular cell type under particular conditions. The possibility also exists, of course, that IFN-β_2 could be induced via different pathways by different agents. Indeed, there is evidence that TNF and IL-1 enhance IFN-β_2 gene transcription via different mechanisms (Walther *et al.*, 1987).

The finding that TPA-induced differentiation of histiocytic lymphoma-derived cells towards macrophage-like cells is associated with endogenous production of IFN-β (Kimchi *et al.*, 1983; Yarden *et al.*, 1984; Ferbus *et al.*, 1985) may have its explanation in the activation of protein kinase C in these cells.

No information is as yet available on the substrate proteins for C kinase that may play a role in mediating increased expression of the IFN-β_2 gene.

It is important to note that one and the same cytomodulating agent can and commonly does activate more than one signal transduction pathway. In quiescent mouse 3T3 cells, PDGF rapidly increases the concentration of free intracellular Ca^{2+} ($[Ca^{2+}]_i$) (Berridge *et al.*, 1984; Kaibuchi *et al.*, 1986) and at the same time activates protein kinase C (Habenicht *et al.*, 1981; Rozengurt *et al.*, 1983; Blackshear *et al.*, 1985; Kaibuchi *et al.*, 1986). These signal transduction events are followed by an increase in the c-*myc* mRNA level (Kelly *et al.*, 1985; Müller *et al.*, 1984; Kaibuchi *et al.*, 1986). Ca^{2+} ionophores (A23187 and ionomycin, $< 2\mu M$) can increase $[Ca^{2+}]_i$ without stimulating protein kinase C, while protein kinase C activators (1-oleoyl-2-acetylglycerol and TPA) stimulate protein kinase C without increasing $[Ca^{2+}]_i$ (Kaibuchi *et al.*, 1986). The Ca^{2+} ionophores and the protein kinase C-activating agents increase c-*myc* mRNA levels in an additive manner. In cells in which protein kinase C has been down-regulated by prolonged incubation with phorbol 12,13-dibutyrate, c-*myc* levels cannot be increased with 1-oleyl-2-acetylglycerol or 12-*O*-tetradecanoylphorbol 13-acetate, but can be increased with Ca^{2+} ionophores. These findings indicate that one and the same gene, the c-*myc* proto-oncogene, can be activated via two distinct second messenger pathways.

Experiments with PDGF and TPA have further demonstrated that activation of transcription of different genes in response to a cytomodulating agent may be mediated via different pathways. PDGF activates the transcription not only of c-*myc* but also of c-*fos*, JE and KC genes and a *fos*-related gene (r-*fos*), among others (Hall and Stiles, 1986). In addition to activating c-*myc*, TPA also induces c-*fos*, but it causes transcriptional repression of JE, KC and r-*fos*. Thus, when PDGF induces JE, KC and r-*fos*, it is likely to be doing so via a pathway other than the diacylglycerol-protein kinase C pathway.

It is noteworthy that the 5′-flanking region of the IFN-β_2 gene contains nucleotide sequence elements that have similarities with the serum-responsive element in c-*fos* (Walther *et al.*, 1987).

There is evidence which indicates that IFN-α and -γ species can also be induced endogenously (Lebon *et al.*, 1981, 1982; Bocci *et al.*, 1984; Belardelli *et al.*, 1984). It remains to be determined which signal transduction pathways operate in the endogenous activation of IFN-α and -γ genes.

Some general statements appear to be in order. If two cytokines that induce gene expression in a given cell type activate the same signal transduction pathways in a unique manner and neither of them activates any other signal transduction pathways, then it may be expected that the two cytokines would induce the expression of the same gene(s). If, however, the two cytokines share signal transduction pathways, but do not activate the pathways exactly the same way or also activate one or more other, distinctive pathways, then the two cytokines may induce some genes in common, but, in addition, may induce or fail to induce certain other genes. Finally, if two cytokines use different signal transduction pathways in a given cell type, they may induce the expression of different genes, but they could also induce some genes in common, as induction of one and the same gene could come about via the activation of different signal transduction pathways. There are many possibilities for diversity in signal transduction pathways, as was discussed in Section III-A.

Protein binding to and dissociation from specific 5′-flanking or promoter regions are likely to be mechanisms for the regulation of the activity of IFN genes. The question is how the activation of a particular signal pathway leads to changes in the binding of specific regulatory proteins to one or more IFN genes.

B Pathways for Mediating IFN Action

The diacylglycerol-protein kinase C pathway is one of the pathways that may mediate IFN action on cells through the activation of IFN-inducible genes. Results of recent studies with IFN-α, -β and -γ species in human fibroblasts, IFN-α and -β species in lymphoblastoid cells, and IFN-γ in macrophages, have provided evidence of the activation of the diacylglycerol-protein kinase C pathway by IFNs (Yap *et al.*, 1986a, b; Hamilton *et al.*, 1985). At least in Daudi cells, IFN-α or -β does not appear to cause an increase in free intracellular Ca^{2+} concentration (Nachshen *et al.*, 1986; Yap *et al.*, 1986a), which, if characteristic of IFN action in a variety of cell types, is a potentially important facet of the transduction of the IFN signal. The activation of the diacylglycerol-protein kinase C pathway correlates with the biological effects of IFNs on these cells. It should be possible, with the aid of synthetic diacylglycerols and by other means, to determine whether the activation of the transcription of IFN-inducible genes can be mediated via the diacylglycerol-protein kinase C pathway. This would, of course, not prove that they are so mediated in the cell. Studies with variant cell lines are necessary. It is such studies that have indicated that cAMP may be required to mediate the antiproliferative action of IFN in macrophage-like cells (Schneck *et al.*, 1982).

When cells that have the potential to differentiate are treated with a phorbol ester such as TPA, differentiation will often be either facilitated or blocked (reviewed in Darnell *et al.*, 1986). IFNs, like TPA, can either facilitate or block differentiation. It has not been rigorously shown that the effects of TPA on differentiation are exclusively mediated via activation of protein kinase C, and they may not all be. Some of the TPA effects could also be due to perturbation of cell membranes, generation of superoxide, or other actions of TPA, as TPA is not always used at the low concentration (10 ng/ml or less) at which its protein kinase C-activating effect is thought to be selective (Nishizuka, 1984). However, if the activation of protein kinase C does play an important role in TPA's effects on differentiation, and if IFN action in a number of cell systems is mediated at least in significant part via diacylglycerol production and protein kinase C activation, then the following questions arise: (1) What are the specific molecular mechanisms that underlie the enhancement versus the inhibition of differentiation? (2) Is the type of response observed a function of the species of origin of the cells, the cell type, or stage of differentiation? (3) Do given cells respond in a particular way because TPA or IFN induces the synthesis of distinctive proteins or because given cells respond uniquely to one or more of the proteins that TPA or IFN may induce in a variety of different kinds of cells? (4) If different IFN-α or -β species have qualitatively different effects on the differentiation of given cells, how are they brought about?

A major problem will continue to be the matter of linking specific IFN-induced proteins to the biological effects of IFNs on cells, such as inhibition of cell proliferation, motility, or transformation, and enhancement or inhibition of cell differentiation. What would be useful are cell mutants that lack or are deficient in an inducible protein or a group of such proteins and which prove unresponsive to a particular biological effect of IFN. Although several of the IFN-induced proteins have been identified, the precise role of proteins such as the double-stranded RNA-dependent 2′,5′A synthetase and protein kinase, and the class I and class II HLA antigens, in mediating the biological effects of IFNs on cells is not clear.

IFNs are capable of exerting some effects on cells very rapidly (e.g. the suppression of synthesis of growth factor-induced proteins in quiescent fibroblasts and receptor redistribution (capping) in lymphocytes or lymphoblastoid cells), whereas other IFN effects take considerable time to develop (e.g. increase organization of actin-containing microfilaments in fibroblasts and HeLa tumour cells and down-regulation of insulin receptors in Daudi cells). In some exponentially dividing cell populations IFNs cause a considerable decrease in the rate of cell proliferation within 24 hours (e.g. in HeLa cells), but in others a longer time is required (e.g. Daudi cells). This may reflect differences in the mechanisms by which IFNs inhibit cell proliferation-related processes in different cell types. The assumption is unwarranted that a single cascade pathway underlies all of the phenotypic changes ultimately displayed by IFN-treated cells.

IFN treatment of cells can result in marked and selective inhibition of the expression of cellular genes, as documented in studies on cell proliferation, differentiation, and transformation. Do IFNs block the mechanisms that drive or enable the expression of these genes (e.g. some step in the signal transduction pathway used by a growth or differentiation factor) or do IFNs act through IFN-inducible gene repressors? Further work in a variety of systems should reveal the answers. What is clear is that, in time, IFNs can bring about changes in processes of fundamental importance to the cell. For example, treatment of HeLa cells for 24 hours with IFN-β markedly decreases the ability of the cells to respond to the lectin concanavalin A with increased calcium exchange and uptake (Pfeffer and Tamm, 1986). Such an impairment in the calcium response mechanism could affect the ability of cells to respond to growth factors and peptide hormones. The decreased abundance of insulin receptors on IFN-α treated IFN-sensitive Daudi cells has broad implications for the functioning of the cells and is associated with decreased proliferation of the cells (Pfeffer *et al.*, 1986, 1987b). Not all of the IFN-induced phenotypic changes in cells are likely to be due to suppression of the expression of genes.

It is an open question as to how IFNs can alter the plasma membrane structure (lipid bilayer fluidity) and function (receptor redistribution) within a short time (30 minutes) and what the biological significance of these effects is.

C IFNs as Cytokines

Endogenous IFNs play varied roles in the normal processes of cell proliferation (negative effect) and differentiation (positive and possibly negative effects). TNF has a mitogenic effect on quiescent human fibroblasts (Sugarman *et al.*, 1985; Vilček *et al.*, 1986), but at the same time it induces IFN-β_2, which counteracts the mitogenic effect of TNF by negative feedback (Kohase *et al.*, 1986). IFN-β_2 mRNA is constitutively expressed in human fibroblasts at a low level, and it is also expressed in several other types of cells, including T cells (Hirano *et al.*, 1986) and monocytes (Vaquero *et al.*, 1986). IFN-β_2 induces B cell differentiation into antibody-producing cells (Hirano *et al.*, 1985; Kishimoto, 1985). Being induced by various cytokines in a wide variety of cell types, IFN-β_2 can be expected to play varied roles, depending on the tissue in which enhanced production occurs and the circumstances under which its production is enhanced. The low levels of constitutively produced IFN-β_2 could also have physiological significance. The fact that sections of the amino acid sequences of IFN-β_2 and the colony-stimulating factor G-CSF are similar and contain four matching cysteine residues may also be important (Hirano *et al.*, 1986). Some of the broader aspects of IFN-β_2 are discussed in detail elsewhere (Sehgal *et al.*, 1987a; Vilček, 1987). A number of other IFN-β species remain to be characterized in detail, including the product of the IFN-β_3 locus located on human chromosome 2 (Slate and Ruddle, 1979; Sagar *et al.*, 1982, 1984; Sehgal *et al.*, 1982a; May *et al.*, 1985; Resnitzky *et al.*, 1986).

IFN-α can act as a differentiation signal for T lymphocytes and cause the acquisition of specific lytic function (Chen *et al.*, 1986a). IFN-α induces two successive rearrangements in the gene for the T cell receptor α-chain (Chen *et al.*, 1986b).

The finding of endogenous IFN-α or -β species in a variety of normal situations and pathological conditions is in and of itself important, and the importance of such findings is augmented by evidence which suggests that the IFNs play a role in host defence against infections and tumours as well as in regulated tissue growth or maintenance.

Like cytokines, IFNs belong to a multicomponent regulatory system within which the interactions of the components are highly complex (Kohase *et al.*, 1986, 1987a). A cytokine may antagonize, enhance or mediate the actions of another cytokine. Different IFNs can undoubtedly play different roles in various physiological settings. One and the same IFN can probably also play different roles in different settings, as illustrated by the fact that IFN-β_2, which suppresses the proliferation of human fibroblasts (Kohase *et al.*, 1986), acts as a growth factor in murine hybridoma/plasmacytoma lines (Van Damme *et al.*, 1987). This is not without precedent as TNF and tumour growth factor (TGF)-β also suppress or stimulate cell proliferation, depending on the cell type (reviewed in Sehgal *et al.*, 1987a).

IFNs are regulated not only at the level of production but also at the level of action. Of particular interest and importance from the viewpoint of IFN function in regulating physiological processes and responses is the fact that cell growth factors can counteract IFN action.

X REMARKS

It is evident that IFNs are important cellular regulatory molecules, as was anticipated some years ago (Gresser, 1977).

Molecular biological tools are in hand to define precisely how IFN genes and the IFN-inducible or IFN-suppressible genes are regulated at the chromosomal level. Critical aspects of the operation of the cytokine network to which IFNs belong can be defined by establishing the signal transduction mechanisms involved in the activation of the expression of the various cytokines by other cytokines and external stimuli. How transduced signals are transmitted to the nucleus is an area that is still poorly understood. Induction of IFN-β_2 expression is an example of a system that lends itself very well to studies of this mechanism, which is itself of broad interest in cell biology.

Knowledge of IFN-inducible proteins is continuing to grow rapidly, and with extensive use of cell mutants it should become possible to link a variety of IFN-induced proteins to specific biological effects of IFNs. It will then be possible to define how IFN-induced proteins exert their effects: by acting as enzymes, gene activators, enhancers, or repressors, or in some other way. A number of the IFN-inducible proteins are no longer to be thought of as proteins appearing or functioning in only very restricted circumstances. The 2′,5′A synthetase system is as much part of the general equipment of the cells as are the major histocompatibility antigens, and will need to be understood in the broader context.

Receptor up- or down-regulation is emerging as one of the means through which cytokine action can be affected.

Much remains to be learned about the precise role in cell physiology of the cellular proto-oncogene products, whose synthesis can be suppressed by IFNs. A better understanding of a number of aspects of IFN action depends directly on this. Clarification of how the expression of oncogenes can lead to neoplastic transformation, and how putative anti-oncogene products can suppress this process, may help in understanding the anti-oncogenic action of IFNs.

The IFN system is a regulatory system, and when a component of the system becomes strongly activated powerful mechanisms appear to exist to limit the activated state.

ACKNOWLEDGEMENTS

We thank Dr Lester T. May for extensive contributions over the years to various aspects of our research, and Doctors Masayoshi Kohase and Jan Vilček for collaboration in the recent developments in the IFN-β_2 area. We wish to thank Ms Celia K. Graham for expert preparation and Ms Toyoko Kikuchi for critical reading of this manuscript.

Work from our laboratory described in this article was supported by USPHS Research Grants CA18608 from the National Cancer Institute, AI16262 from the National Institute of Allergy and Infectious Diseases, and GM46716 from the National Institute of General Medical Sciences; by USPHS Program Project Grant CA18213 from the National Cancer Institute, and the National Research Service Award AI07233; and by a grant from the Elsa M. Pardee Foundation and a contract from the Foundation for Cancer Research. Dr L. M. Pfeffer is a Leukemia Society of America Scholar and Dr P. B. Sehgal is an Established Investigator of the American Heart Association.

REFERENCES

Aderka, D., Levo, Y., Rahmany, R., Mory, Y., Vaks, B., Horovitz, O., Doerner, T., Shoham, J., Wallach, D. and Revel, M. (1985). *Israel J. Med. Sci.* **21**, 977–981.

Aguet, M. (1980). *Nature (London)* **284**, 459–461.

Anderson, P., Yip, Y. K. and Vilček, J. (1982). *J. Biol. Chem.* **257**, 11301–11304.

Armelin, H. A., Armelin, M. C. S., Kelly, K., Stewart, T., Leder, P., Cochran, B. H. and Stiles, C. D. (1984). *Nature (London)* **310**, 655–660.

Auböck, J., Niederweiser, D., Romani, N., Fritsch, P. and Huber, C. (1985). *Arch. Dermatol. Res.* **4**, 270–275.

Bachwich, P. R., Chensue, S. W., Larrick, J. W. and Kunkel, S. L. (1986). *Biochem. Biophys. Res. Comm.* **136**, 94–101.

Baglioni, C., Branca, A. A., d'Alessandro, S. B., Hossenslop, D. and Chadha K. C. (1982). *Virol.* **122**, 202–206.

Balkwill, F. and Taylor-Papadimitriou, J. (1978). *Nature (London)* **274**, 798–800.

Baron, S. (1967). *In* "Interferons" (N. B. Finter, ed.), pp. 268–313. North-Holland Publishing Co., Amsterdam.

Bartram, C. R., de Klein, A., Hagemeijer, A., van Agthoven, T., van Kessel, A.-D., Bootsma, D., Grosveld, G., Ferguson-Smith, M. A., Davies, T., Stone, M., Heisterkamp, N., Stephenson, J. R. and Groffen, J. (1983). *Nature (London)* **306**, 277–280.

Baserga, R. (1985). *In* "The Biology of Cell Reproduction", pp. 251, Harvard University Press, Cambridge.

Basham, T. Y., Nickoloff, B. J., Merigan, T. C. and Morhenn, V. B. (1985). *J. Interferon Res.* **1**, 23–32.

Belardelli, F., Vignaux, F., Proietti, E. and Gresser, I. (1984). *Proc. Natl Acad. Sci. USA* **81**, 602–606.

Benech, P., Mory, Y., Revel, M. and Chebath, J. (1985a). *EMBO J.* **4**, 2249–2256.

Benech, P., Merlin, G., Revel, M. and Chebath, J. (1985b). *Nucleic Acids Res.* **13**, 1267–1281.

Berman, B., Duncan, M. R., Smith, R., Ziboh, V. A. and Palladino, M. (1985). *J. Invest. Dermatol.* **1**, 54–58.

Berridge, M. J. and Irvine, R. F. (1984). *Nature (London)* **312**, 315–321.

Berridge, M. J., Heslop, J. P., Irvine, R. F. and Brown, K. D. (1984). *Biochem. J.* **222**, 195–201.

Berridge, M. J., Heslop, J. P., Irvine, R. F. and Brown, K. D. (1985). *Biochem. Soc. Trans.* **13**, 67–71.

Besançon, F., Bourgeade, M. F. and Testa, U. (1985). *J. Biol. Chem.* **260**, 13074–13080.

Besterman, J. M., Duronio, V. and Cuatrecasas, P. (1986). *Proc. Natl Acad. Sci. USA* **83**, 6785–6789.

Bhat, R. A. and Thimmappaya, B. (1983). *Proc. Natl Acad. Sci. USA* **80**, 4789–4793.

Bhat, R. A. and Thimmappaya, B. (1985). *J. Virology* **56**, 750–756.

Billard, C., Ferbus, D., Kolb, J. P., Rosa, F., Perrot, J. Y., Merlin, G., Janiaud, P., Raynaud, N., Thang, M. N., Fellous, M. *et al.* (1986). *Ann. Inst. Pasteur Immunol.* **3**, 259–272.

Billiau, A. (1986). *Nature (London)* **324**, 415.

Blackshear, P. J., Witters, L. A., Girard, P. R., Kuo, J. F. and Quamo, S. N. (1985). *J. Biol. Chem.* **269**, 13304–13315.

Blair, D. G., Oskarsson, M., Wood, T. G. and McClements, W. L. (1981). *Science* **212**, 941–942.

Bocci, V., Muscettola, M., Paulesu, L. and Grasso, G. (1984). *J. Gen. Virol.* **65**, 101–108.

Boumpas, D. T., Hooks, J. J., Popovic, M., Tsokos, G. C. and Mann, D. L. (1985). *J. Clin. Immunol.* **5**, 340–344.

Bourgeade, M. F., Rousset, S., Paulen, D. and Chaney, C. (1981). *J. Interferon Res.* **1**, 323–332.

Bradley, E. C. and Ruscetti, F. W. (1981). *Cancer Res.* **41**, 244–249.

Branca, A. A. and Baglioni, C. (1981). *Nature (London)* **294**, 768–770.

Branca, A. A., Faltynek, C. R., D'Allessandro, S. B. and Baglioni, C. (1982). *J. Biol. Chem.* **257**, 13291–13296.

Brennan, M. B. and Stark, G. R. (1983). *Cell* **33**, 811–816.

Brouty-Boyé, D. and Zetter, B. R. (1980). *Science* **208**, 516–518.

Brouty-Boyé, D., Cheng, Y.-S. E. and Chen, L. B. (1981). *Cancer Res.* **41**, 4174–4184.

Brouty-Boyé, D., Mogensen, K. E. and Gresser, I. (1985). *Eur. J. Cancer Clin. Oncol.* **21**, 507–514.

Brouty-Boyé, D., Wybier-Franqui, J., Nardeux, P., Daya-Grosjean, L., Andeol, Y. and Suarez, H. G. (1986). *J. Interferon Res.* **6**, 461–478.

Broxmeyer, H. E., Bognacki, J., Ralph, P., Dorner, M. H., Lu, L. and Castro-Malaspina, H. (1982). *Blood* **60**, 595–607.

Burrone, O. R. and Milstein, C. (1982). *EMBO J.* **1**, 345–349.

Burrone, O. R., Kefford, R. F., Gilmore, D. and Milstein, G. (1985). *EMBO J.* **1**, 2855–2860.

Capobianchi, M. R., Ameglio, F., Tosi, R. and Dolei, A. (1985). *Hum. Immunol.* **1**, 1–11.

Carrel, S., Schmidt-Kessen, A. and Giuffrie, L. (1985). *Eur. J. Immunol.* **2**, 118–123.

Carter, W. A., Strayer, D. R., Hubbell, H. R. and Brodsky, I. (1985). *J. Biol. Res. Mod.* **4**, 495–502.

Chatterjee, S., Cheung, H. E. and Hunter, E. (1982). *Proc. Natl Acad. Sci. USA* **79**, 835–839.

Chebath, J., Benech, P. and Revel, M. (1986). *J. Interferon Res.* **6**, Supplement 1, 21.

Chebath, J., Benech, P. and Revel, M. (1987). *J. Biol. Chem.* **262,** 3852–3857.

Chen, B. D.-M. (1986). *J. Immunol.* **136**, 174–180.

Chen, L. K., Tourvieille, B., Burns, G. F., Bach, F. H., Mathieu-Mahul, D., Sasportes, M., Bensussan, A. (1986a). *Eur. J. Immunol.* **16**, 767–770.

Chen, L. K., Mathieu-Mahul, Bach F. H., Dausset, J., Bensussan, A. and Sasportes, M. (1986b). *Proc. Natl Acad. Sci. USA* **83**, 4887–4889.

Cioé, L., O'Brien, T. G. and Diamond, L. (1980). *Cell Biol. Int. Rep.* **4**, 255–264.

Cleveland, D. W., Lopata, M. A., MacDonald, J., Cowan, N. J., Rutter, W., Land, H. and Kirschner, M. W. (1980). *Cell* **20**, 95–105.

Cleveland, D. W., Lopata, M. A., Sherline, P. and Kirschner, M. W. (1981). *Cell* **25**, 537–546.

Cochran, B. H., Reffel, A. C. and Stiles, C. D. (1983). *Cell* **33**, 939–947.

Collins, T., Lapierre, L. A., Fiers, W., Strominger, J. L. and Pober, J. S. (1986). *Proc. Natl Acad. Sci. USA* **83**, 446–450.

Connolly, T. M., Lawing, W. J. Jr and Majerus, P. W. (1986). *Cell* **46**, 951–958.

Content, J., De Wit, L., Poupart, P., Opdenakker, G., Van Damme, J. and Billiau, A. (1985). *Eur. J. Biochem.* **152**, 253–257.

Cooper, J. A., Bowen-Pope, D. F., Raines, E., Ross, R. and Hunter, T. (1982). *Cell* **31**, 263–273.

Coughlin, S. R., Lee, W. M. F., Williams, P. W., Giels, G. M. and Williams, L. T. (1985). *Cell* **43**, 243–251.

Dani, Ch., Mechti, N., Piechaczyk, Lebleu, B., Jeanteur, Ph. and Blanchard, J. M. (1985). *Proc. Natl Acad. Sci. USA* **82**, 4896–4899.

Daniel, L. W., Waite, M. and Wykle, R. L. (1986). *J. Biol. Chem.* **261**, 9128–9132.

Darnell, J., Lodish, H. and Baltimore, D. (1986). *In* "Molecular Cell Biology", p. 1187. Scientific American Books, New York.

Dayton, E. T., Matsumoto-Kobayashi, M., Perussia, B. and Trinchieri, G. (1985). *Blood* **66**, 583–594.

De Mayer-Guignard, J. and De Mayer, E. (1985). *Interferon* **6**, 69–91.

Der, C. J. and Cooper, G. M. (1983). *Cell* **32**, 201–208.

Diaz-Espada, F., Milstein, C. and Secher, D. (1986). *Cell Immunol.* **100**, 331–339.

Dinarello, C. A., Cannon, J. G., Wolff, S. M., Bernheim, H. A., Beutler, B., Cerami, A., Figari, I., Palladino, M. A. and O'Connor, J. V. (1986). *J. Exp. Med.* **163**, 1433–1450.

Doyle, A, Martin, W. J., Funa, K., Gazdar, A., Carney, D., Martin, S. E., Linnoila, I., Cuttiıta, F., Mulshine, J., Bunn, P. and Minna, J. (1985). *J. Exp. Med.* **161**, 1135–1151.

Dron, M. and Tovey, M. G. (1983). *J. Gen. Virol.* **64**, 2641–2647.

Dron, M., Tovey, M. G. and Eid, P. (1985). *J. Gen. Virol.* **66**, 787–795.

Dron, M., Modjtahedi, N., Brison, O. and Tovey, M. G. (1986). *Mol. Cell. Biol.* **6**, 1374–1378.

Einat, M., Resnitzky, D. and Kimchi, A. (1985a). *Proc. Natl Acad. Sci. USA* **82**, 7608–7612.

Einat, M., Resnitzky, D. and Kimchi, A. (1985b). *Nature (London)* **313**, 597–600.

Erikson, J., Ar-Rushdi, A. A., Drwinga, H. L., Nowell, P. C. and Croce, C. M. (1983). *Proc. Natl Acad. Sci. USA* **80**, 820–824.

Faltynek, C. R., Branca, A. A., McCandless, S. and Baglioni, C. (1983). *Proc. Natl Acad. Sci. USA* **80**, 3269–3273.

Farese, R. V., Davis, J. S., Barnes, D. E., Standaert, M. L., Babischkin, J. S., Hock, R., Rosie, N. K. and Pollet, R. J. (1985). *Biochem. J.* **231**, 269–278.

Fellous, M., Nir, U., Wallach, D., Merlin, G., Rubinstein, M. and Revel, M. (1982a). *Proc. Natl Acad. Sci. USA* **79**, 3082—3086.

Fellous, A., Ginzburg, I. and Littauer, U. Z. (1982b). *EMBO J.* **1**, 835–839.

Ferbus, D., Testa, U., Titeux, M., Louache, F. and Thang, M. N. (1985). *Mol. Cell. Biochem.* **67**, 125–133.

Fisher, P. B., Mufson, R. A. and Weinstein, I. B. (1981). *Biochem. Biophys. Res. Commun.* **100**, 823–830.

Fisher, P. B., Miranda, A. F., Babiss, L. E., Pestka, S. and Weinstein, I. B. (1983). *Proc. Natl Acad. Sci. USA* **80**, 2961–2965.

Fisher, P.B., Prignoli, D.R., Mermo, H. Jr, Weinstein, I. B. and Pestka, S. (1985). *J. Interferon Res.* **5**, 11–22.

Fraser, N. W., Sehgal, P. B. and Darnell, J. E. (1978). *Nature (London)* **272**, 590–593.

Fraser, N. W., Sehgal, P. B. and Darnell, J. E. (1979). *Proc. Natl Acad. Sci. USA* **76**, 2571–2575.

Friedman, R. L. and Stark, G. R. (1985). *Nature (London)* **314**, 837–839.

Friedman, R. L., Manly, S. P., McMahon, M., Kerr, I. M. and Stark, G. R. (1984). *Cell* **38**, 745–755.

Friedman-Einat, M., Revel, M. and Kimchi, A. (1982). *Mol. Cell. Biol.* **2**, 1472–1480.

Fujita, T., Ohno, S., Yasumitsu, H. and Taniguchi, T. (1985). *Cell* **41**, 489–496.

Furth, M. E., Davis, L. J., Fleurdelys, B. and Scolnick, E. M. (1982). *J. Virol.* **43**, 294–305.

Fuse, A., Mahmud, I. and Kuwata, T. (1982). *Cancer Res.* **42**, 3209–3214.

Gal, S. and Gottesman, M. M. (1986). *J. Biol. Chem.* **261**, 1760–1765.

Gallien-Lartigue, I., Carrez, D., De Maeyer, E. and De Maeyer-Guignard, J. (1980). *Science* **209**, 292–293.

Gallien-Lartigue, O., De Maeyer-Guignard, J., Carrez, D. and De Maeyer, E. (1985). *J. Interferon Res.* **5**, 347–354.

Garcia-Blanco, M. A., Ghosh, P. K., Jayaram, B. M., Ivory, S., Lebowitz, P. and Lengyel, P. (1985). *J. Virol.* **53**, 893–898.

Garson, D., Dokhela, M. C., Wakasugi, H., Mishal, Z. and Tursz, T. (1985). *Hematol.* **13**, 885–890.

Gastl, G., Marth, C., Leiter, E., Gattringer, C., Mayer, I., Daxenbichler, G., Flener, R. and Huber, C. (1985). *Cancer Res.* **7**, 2957–2961.

Goodbourn, S., Zinn, K. and Maniatis, T. (1985). *Cell* **41**, 509–520.
Goodbourn, S., Burstein, H. and Maniatis, T. (1986). *Cell* **45**, 601–610.
Gottesman, M. M. (1978). *Proc. Natl Acad. Sci. USA* **75**, 2767–2771.
Gottesman, M. M. and Sobel, M. E. (1980). *Cell* **19**, 449–455.
Grant, S., Bhalla, K., Weinstein, B., Pestka, S., Mileno, M. D. and Fisher, P. B. (1985). *Biochem. Biophys. Res. Commun.* **130**, 379–388.
Green, S. H. and Greene, L. A. (1986). *J. Biol. Chem.* **261**, 15316–15326.
Greenberg, M. E. and Ziff, E. B. (1984). *Nature (London)* **311**, 433–438.
Greiner, J. W., Fisher, P. B, Pestka, S. and Schlom, J. (1986). *Cancer Res.* **46**, 4984–4990.
Gresser, I. (1977). *Cell. Immunol.* **34**, 406–415.
Gresser, I., Bourali, C., Levy, J. P., Fontaine-Brouty-Boyé, D. and Thomas, M. T. (1969). *Proc. Natl Acad. Sci. USA* **63**, 51–57.
Gresser, I., Belardelli, F., Maury, C., Maunory, M.-T. and Tovey, M. G. (1983). *J. Exp. Med.* **158**, 2095–2107.
Gresser, I., Vignaux, F., Belardelli, F., Tovey, M. G. and Maunoury, M.-T. (1985). *J. Virol.* **53**, 221–227.
Grossberg, S. E. and Keay, S. (1980). *Ann. NY Acad. Sci.* **350**, 294–300.
Grossberg, S. E. and Sabran, J. L. (1982). *Tex. Rep. Biol. Med.* **41**, 332–335.
Grove, G. L., Anderton, R. L. and Smith, J. G. Jr (1976). *J. Invest. Dermatol.* **66**, 236–238.
Habenicht, A. J. R., Glomset, J. A., King, W. C., Nist, C., Mitchell, C. D. and Ross, R. (1981). *J. Biol. Chem.* **256**, 12329–12335.
Haddada, H., Lewis, A. M., Sogn, J. A., Coligan, J. E., Cook, J. L., Walker, T. A. and Levine, A. S. (1986). *Proc. Natl Acad. Sci. USA* **83**, 9684–9688.
Haegeman, G., Content, J., Volckaert, G., Derynck, R., Tavernier, J. and Fiers, W. (1986). *Eur. J. Biochem.* **159**, 625–632.
Hall, D. J. and Stiles, C. D. (1986). *J. Cell Biol.* Abstr. **103**, 150a.
Hamilton, T. A., Becton, D. L., Somers, S. D., Gray, P. W. and Adams, D. O. (1985). *J. Biol. Chem.* **260**, 1378–1381.
Hannigan, G. E. and Williams, B. R. G. (1986). *EMBO J.* **5**, 1607–1613.
Hannigan, G. E., Lau, A. G. and Williams, B. R. (1986). *Eur. J. Biochem.* **157**, 187–193.
Hassan, Y., Huleihel, M., Priel, E., Wolfson, M. and Aboud, M. (1985). *Carcinogenesis* **12**, 1787–1790.
Havell, E. A. and Vilček, J. (1972). *Antimicrob. Agents Chemother.* **2**, 476–484.
Hayashi, H., Tanaka, K., Jay, F., Khoury, G. and Jay, G. (1985). *Cell* **43**, 263–267.
Hesketh, T. R., Moore, J. P., Morris, J. D. H., Taylor, M. V., Rogers, J., Smith, G. A. and Metcalf, J. C. (1985). *Nature (London)* **313,** 481–484.
Hicks, N. J., Morris, A. G. and Burke, D. C. (1981). *J. Cell Sci.* **49**, 225–236.
Hirano, T., Taga, T., Nakano, N., Yasukawa, K., Kashiwamura, S., Shimizu, K., Nakajima, A K., Pyun, K. H. and Kishimoto, T. (1985). *Proc. Natl Acad. Sci. USA* **82**, 5490–5494.
Hirano, T., Yasukawa, K., Harada, H., Taga, T., Watanabe, Y., Matsuda, T., Kashiwamura, S., Nakajima, K., Koyama, K., Iwamatsu, A., Tsunasawa S., Sakiyama, F., Matsui, H., Takahara, Y., Taniguchi, T. and Kishimoto, T. (1986). *Nature (London)* **324**, 73–76.
Hirasawa, K. and Nishizuka, Y. (1985). *Ann. Rev. Pharmacol. Toxicol.* **25**, 147–170.
Holt, J. T., Venkat Gopal, T., Moulton, A. D. and Nienhuis, A. W. (1986). *Proc. Natl Acad. Sci. USA* **83**, 4794–4798.
Hovanessian, A. G., Meurs, E., Laurent, A. G. and Svab, J. (1986). *In* "UCLA Symposia: Interferon as Cell Growth and Antitumour Factors" (R. M. Friedman,

T. Sreevalsan and T. Merigan, eds). UCLA Symp. on Molecular and Cellular Biology, Vol. 50, pp. 49–66. A. R. Liss, New York.

Hovi, T., Lehto, V. P. and Virtanen, I. (1985). *Exp. Cell Res.* **159**, 305–312.

Hubbell, H. R. (1986). *Int. J. Cancer* **37**, 359–365.

Hubbell, H. R., Lliu, R.-S. and Maxwell, B. L. (1984). *Cancer Res.* **44**, 3252–3257.

Hubbell, H. R., Kvalnes-Krick, K., Carter, W. A. and Strayer, D. R. (1985). *Cancer Res.* **45**, 2481–2486.

Huygen, K. and Verschueren, R. (1986). *J. Interferon Res.* **6**, Supplement 1, 71.

Ilson, D. H., Torrence, P. F. and Vilček, J. (1986). *J. Interferon Res.* **6**, 5–12.

Inagaki, M., Kawamoto, S. and Hidaka, H. (1984). *J. Biol. Chem.* **259**, 14321–14323.

Inglot, A. D., Oleszak, E. and Kisielow, B. (1980). *Arch. Virol.* **63**, 291–296.

Jacobs, A. D., Champlin, R. E. and Golde, D. W. (1985). *Blood* **65**, 1017–1020.

Jennings, S. R., Rice, P. R., Koszewski, E. D., Anderson, R. W., Thompson, D. L. and Tevethia, S. S. (1985). *J. Virol.* **56**, 757–766.

Jonak, G. J. and Knight, E. (1984). *Proc. Natl Acad. Sci. USA* **81**, 1747–1750.

Kaczmarek, L., Hyland, J, Watt, R., Rosenberg, M. and Baserga, R. (1985). *Science* **228**, 1313–1315.

Kaibuchi, K., Tsuda, T., Kikuchi, A., Tanimoto, T., Yamashita, T. and Takai, Y. (1986). *J. Biol. Chem.* **261**, 1187–1192.

Keay, S. and Grossberg, S. E. (1980). *Proc. Natl Acad. Sci. USA* **77**, 4099–4013.

Kelly, K., Cochran, B. H., Stiles, C. D. and Leder, P. (1983). *Cell* **35**, 603–610.

Kelly, J. M., Gilbert, C. S., Stark, G. R. and Kerr, I. M. (1985). *Eur. J. Biochem.* **153**, 367–371.

Kikutani, H., Taga, T., Akira, S., Kishi, H., Miki, Y., Saiki, O., Yamamura, Y. and Kishimoto, T. (1985). *J. Immunol.* **134**, 990–995.

Kimchi, A., Shure, H., Lapidot, Y., Rapoport, S., Panet, A. and Revel, M. (1981). *FEBS Lett.* **134**, 212–216.

Kimchi, A., Bendori, R., Einat, M., Yarden, A., Resnitzky, D. and Gottlieb, H. (1983). *In* "Biology of the Interferon System 1983" (E. De Maeyer and H. Schellekens, eds), pp. 83–90. Elsevier Science Publishers, Amsterdam.

Kishimoto, T. (1985). *Ann. Rev. Immunol.* **3**, 133–157.

Kishimoto, T. and Ishizaka, K. (1973). *J. Immunol.* **111**, 1194–1205.

Kitajewski, J., Schneider, R. J., Safer, B., Munemitsu, S. M., Samuel, C. E., Thimmaapaya, B. and Shenk, T. (1986a). *Cell* **45**, 195–200.

Kitajewski, J., Schneider, R. J., Safer, B. and Slenk, T. (1986b). *Mol. Cell. Biol.* **6**, 4493–4498.

Klein, G. and Klein, E. (1985). *Nature (London)* **315**, 190–195.

Kloetzer, W., Kurzrock, R., Smith, L., Talpaz, M., Spiller, M., Gutterman, J. and Arlinghaus, R. (1985). *Virology* **140**, 230–238.

Knight, E., Anton, E. D., Fahey, D., Friedland, B. K. and Jonak, G. J. (1985). *Proc. Natl Acad. Sci. USA* **82**, 1151–1154.

Kohase, M., Henriksen-DeStefano, D., May, L. T., Vilček, J. and Sehgal, P. B. (1986). *Cell* **45**, 659–666.

Kohase, M., May, L. T., Tamm, I., Vilček, J. and Sehgal, P. B. (1987a). *Mol. Cell. Biol.* **7**, 273–280.

Kohase, M., Henriksen-DeStefano, D., Sehgal, P. B. and Vilček, J. (1987b). *J. Cell. Physiol.* (submitted).

Kohase, M., Tsujimoto, M., May, L. T., Sehgal, P. B. and Vilček, J. (1987c). *In* "The Biology of the Interferon System 1986" (H. Schellekens and K. Cantell, eds). pp. 159–163. Martinus Nijhoff, Boston.

Konopka, J. B., Watanabe, S. M. and Witte, O. N. (1984). *Cell* **37**, 1035–1042.

Krause, D., Panet, A., Arad, G., Dieffenbach, C. W. and Silverman, R. H. (1985). *J. Biol. Chem.* **260**, 9501–9507.

Kruijer, W., Cooper, J. A., Hunter, T. and Verma, I. M. (1984). *Nature (London)* **312**, 711–716.

Kurland, J. I., Bockman, R. S., Broxmeyer, H. E. and Moore, M. A. S. (1978). *Science* **150**, 552.

Kushnaryov, V. M., MacDonald, H. S. Sedmak, J. J. and Grossberg, S. E. (1985). *Proc. Natl Acad. Sci. USA* **82**, 3281–3285.

Larrick, J. W. and Cresswell, P. (1979). *J. Supramol. Struct.* **11**, 579–586.

Lau, L. and Nathans, D. (1985). *EMBO J.* **4**, 3145–3151.

Le, J., Weinstein, D., Gubler, U. and Vilček, J. (1987) *J. Immunol.* **138**, 2137–2142.

Leanderson, T. and Lundgren, E. (1980). *Exp. Cell Res.* **180**, 421–426.

Leanderson, T. and Lundgren, E. (1982). *J. Interferon Res.* **2**, 21–29.

Lebon, P., Girard, S., Thépot, F. and Chany, C. (1981). *C.R. Hedb. Seances Acad. Sci. Ser. III* **293**, 69–71.

Lebon, P., Girard, S., Thépot, F. and Chany, C. (1982). *J. Gen. Virol.* **59**, 393–396.

Leder, P., Battey, J., Lenoir, G., Moulding, C., Murphy, W., Potter, H., Stewart, T. and Taub, R. (1983). *Science* **222**, 765–771.

Lengyel, P. (1982). *Ann. Rev. Biochem.* **51**, 251–282.

Lengyel, P. (1986). *In* "Interferons as Cell Growth Inhibitors and Antitumor Factors" (R. Friedman, T. Merigan and T. Sreevalsan, eds). UCLA Symposia on Molecular and Cellular Biology, New Series, Vol, 50, pp. xxi–xxxviii. A. R. Liss, New York.

Leof, E. B., Wharton, W., Van Wyck, J. J. and Pledger, W. J. (1982). *Exp. Cell. Res.* **141**, 107–115.

Lerner, M. R., Andrews, N. C., Miller, G. and Steitz, J. A. (1981). *Proc. Natl Acad. Sci. USA* **78**, 805–809.

Lin, S. L., Ts'o, P. O. P. and Hollenberg, M. D. (1980). *Biochem. Biophys. Res. Commun.* **96**, 169–174.

Lin, S. L., Greene, J. J., Ts'o, P. O. P. and Carter, W. A. (1982). *Nature (London)* **297**, 417–419.

Lin, S. L., Garber, E. A., Wang, E., Caliguiri, L. A., Schellekens, H., Goldberg, A. R. and Tamm, I. (1983a). *Mol. Cell. Biol.* **3**, 1656–1664.

Lin, S. L., Ts'o, P. O. P. and Hollenberg, M. D. (1983b). *Life Sciences* **32**, 1479–1488.

Lin, S. L., Pledger, W. J. and Tamm, I. (1985). *In* "The Biology of the Interferon System 1985" (W. E. Stewart II and H. Schellekens, eds), pp. 311–314. Elsevier Science Publishers, Amsterdam.

Lin, S. L., Kikuchi, T., Pledger, W. L. and Tamm, I. (1986a). *Science* **233**, 356–359.

Lin, S. L., Schellekens, H. and Tamm, I. (1986b). *J. Interferon Res.* **6**, 563–572.

Lough, J., Keay, S., Sabran, J. L. and Grossberg, S. E. (1982). *Biochem. Biophys. Res. Commun.* **109**, 92–99.

Majerus, P. W., Connolly, T. M., Deckmyn, H., Ross, T. S., Bross, T. E., Ishii, H., Bansal, V. S. and Wilson, D. B. (1986). *Science* **234**, 1519–1526.

Mallucci, L., Rasbridge, S. and Wells, V. (1983). *J. Interferon Res.* **3**, 181–189.

Mallucci, L., Chebath, J., Revel, M., Wells, V. and Benech, P. (1985). *In* "The Interferon System" (F. Dianzani and G. B. Rossi, eds), Serono Symposia Publications, **24**, 165–170. Raven Press, NY.

Mallucci, L., Wells, V., Chebath, J. and Revel, M. (1986). *In* "The Biology of the Interferon System 1985" (W. E. Stewart II and M. Schellekens, eds), pp. 125–130. Elsevier, Amsterdam.

Masuyama, J., Minato, N. and Kano, S. (1986). *J. Clin. Invest.* **77**, 1596–1605.

Matsuyama, M. (1979). *Exp. Cell Res.* **124**, 253–259.

May, L. T., Landsberger, F. R., Inouye, M. and Sehgal, P. B. (1985). *Proc. Natl Acad. Sci. USA* **82**, 4090–4094.

May, L. T., Helfgott, D. C. and Sehgal, P. B. (1986). *Proc. Natl Acad. Sci. USA* **83**, 8957–8961.

Mechti, N., Piechaczyk, J. M., Blanchard, J.-M., Marty, L., Bonnieu, A., Jeanteur, Ph. and Lebleu, B. (1986). *Nucl. Acids Res.* **14**, 9653–9666.

Merlin, G., Chebath, J., Benech, P., Metz, R. and Revel, M. (1983). *Proc. Natl Acad. Sci. USA* **80**, 4904–4908.

Metz, D. H., Levin, M. J. and Oxman, M. N. (1976). *J. Gen. Virol.* **32**, 227–240.

Moehring, J. M., Stinebring, W. R. and Merchant, D. J. (1971). *Applied Microbiol.* **22**, 102–105.

Mogenson, K. E. and Bandu, M.-T. (1983). *Eur. J. Biochem.* **138**, 355–364.

Moore, R. N., Larsen, H. S., Horohov, D. W. and Rouse, B. T. (1984). *Science* **223**, 178–181.

Moore, R. N., Pitruzzello, F. J., Deana, D. G. and Rouse, B. T. (1985). *Lymphokine Res.* **4**, 43–50.

Mozes, L. W. and Defendi, V. (1979). *Virology* **93**, 558–568.

Müller, R., Bravo, R., Burckhardt, J. and Curran, T. (1984). *Nature (London)* **312**, 716–720.

Multhauf, C. and Lough, J. (1986). *J. Cell. Physiol.* **126**, 211–215.

Muraguchi, A., Kishimoto, T., Miki, Y., Kuritani, T., Kaieda, T., Yoshizaki, K. and Yamamura, Y. (1981). *J. Immunol.* **127**, 412–416.

Musgrove, E., Rugg, C., Taylor and Hedley, D. (1984). *J. Cell. Physiol.* **118**, 6–12.

Nachshen, D. A., Pfeffer, L. M. and Tamm, I. (1986). *J. Biol. Chem.* **261**, 15134–15139.

Naka, M., Nishikawa, M., Adelstein, R. S. and Hidaka, H. (1983). *Nature (London)* **306**, 490–492.

Nawroth, P. P., Bank, I., Handley, D., Cassimeris, J., Chess, L. and Stern, D. (1986). *J. Exp. Med.* **163**, 1363–1375.

Neumann, H. A. and Fauser, A. A. (1982). *Exp. Hematol.* **10**, 587–590.

Nir, U., Maroteaux, L., Cohen, B. and Mory, I. (1985). *J. Biol. Chem.* **260**, 14242–14247.

Nishikawa, M., Hidaka, H. and Adelstein, R. S. (1983). *J. Biol. Chem.* **258**, 14069–14072.

Nishizuka, Y. (1984). *Nature (London)* **308**, 693–698.

Okada, M., Sakaguchi, N., Yoshimura, N., Hara, H., Shimizu, K., Yoshida, N., Yoshizaki, K., Kishimoto, S., Yamamura, Y. and Kishimoto, T. (1983). *J. Exp. Med.* **157**, 583–590.

Oladipupo-Williams, C.K., Svet-Moldavskaya, I., Vilček, J., Ohnuma, T. and Holland, J. F. (1981). *Oncology* **38**, 356–360.

Olashaw, N. E. and Pledger, W. J. (1983). *Nature (London)* **306**, 272–274.

Oleszak, E. and Inglot, A. D. (1980). *J. Interferon Res.* **1**, 37–48.

Östlund, L., Einhorn, S., Robèrt, K.-H., Juliusson, G. and Biberfeld, P. (1986). *Blood* **67**, 152–159.

Owen, A. J., Geyer, R. P. and Antoniades, H. N. (1982). *Proc. Natl Acad. Sci. USA* **79**, 3203–3207.

Paez, E. and Esteban, M. (1984). *Virology* **134**, 12–48.

Patton, J. S., Shepard, H. M., Wilking, H., Lewis, G., Aggarwal, B. B., Eessalu, T. E., Gavin, L. A. and Grunfeld, C. (1986). *Proc. Natl Acad. Sci. USA* **83**, 8313–8317.

Paucker, K., Cantell, K. and Henle, W. (1962). *Virology* **17**, 324–334.
Poupart, P., DeWit, L. and Content, J. (1984). *Eur. J. Biochem.* **143**, 15–21.
Pelus, L. M., Broxmeyer, H. E., Kurland, J. I. and Moore, M. A. S. (1979). *J. Exp. Med.* **150**, 277.
Pfeffer, L. M. (1987). *In* "Mechanisms of Interferon Action" (L. M. Pfeffer, ed.). CRC Press. Boca Raton, FL. In press.
Pfeffer, L. M. and Tamm, I. (1982). *J. Interferon Res.* **2**, 431–440.
Pfeffer, L. M. and Tamm, I. (1986). *J. Interferon Res.* **6**, 551–556.
Pfeffer, L. M., Wang, E. and Tamm, I. (1980a). *J. Cell Biol.* **85**, 9–17.
Pfeffer, L. M., Wang, E. and Tamm, I. (1980b). *J. Exp. Med.* **152**, 469–474.
Pfeffer, L. M., Landsberger, F. R. and Tamm, I. (1981). *J. Interferon Res.* **1**, 613–620.
Pfeffer, L. M., Wang, E., Fried, J. and Tamm, I. (1982). *In* "Genetic Expression in the Cell Cycle" (G. M. Padilla and K. S. McCarty, Jr, eds), pp. 289–314. Academic Press, New York.
Pfeffer, L. M., Kwok, B. C. P., Landsberger, F. R. and Tamm, I. (1985). *Proc. Natl Acad. Sci. USA* **82**, 2417–2421.
Pfeffer, L. M., Donner, D. B., Arakawa, T., Stebbing, N. and Tamm, I. (1986). *J. Interferon Res.* **6**, 24.
Pfeffer, L. M., Stebbing, N. and Donner, D. B. (1987a). *Proc. Natl Acad. Sci. USA* (in press).
Pfeffer, L. M., Donner, D. B. and Tamm, I. (1987b). *J. Biol. Chem.* **262,** 3665–3670.
Pickering, L. A. Kronenberg, L. H. and Stewart, W. E. (1980). *Proc. Natl Acad. Sci. USA* **77**, 5938–5942.
Pledger, W. J., Stiles, C. D., Antoniades, H. N. and Scher, C. D. (1977). *Proc. Natl Acad. Sci. USA* **74**, 4481–4485.
Pledger, W. J., Stiles, C. D., Antoniades, H. N. and Scher, C. D. (1978). *Proc. Natl Acad. Sci. USA* **75**, 2839–2843.
Quesada, J. R., Reuben, J. R., Manning, T. J., Hersh, E. M. and Gutterman, J. U. (1984). *New Eng. J. Med.* **310**, 15–18.
Raj, N. B. K. and Pitha, P. M. (1983). *Proc. Natl Acad. Sci. USA* **80**, 3923–3927.
Rasmussen, H. (1986). *New. Eng. J. Med.* **314**, 1164–1170.
Rasmussen, H. and Barret, P. Q. (1984). *Physiol. Rev.* **64**, 938–984.
Resnitzky, D., Yarden, A., Zipori, D. and Kimchi, A. (1986). *Cell* **46**, 31–40.
Revel, M. (1984). *In* "Antiviral Drugs and Interferon" (Y. Becker, ed.), pp. 357–433. Martinus Nijhoff, Boston, MA.
Revel, M. and Michalevicz, R. (1986). *J. Interferon Res.* **6**, Supplement 1, 19.
Revel, M. and Zilberstein, A. (1987). *Nature (London)* **325,** 581–582.
Revel, M., Wallach, D., Merlin, G., Schattner, A., Schmidt, A. and Kimchi, A. (1981). *Meth. Enzymol.* **79**, 149–161.
Rice, A. P. and Kerr, I. M. (1984). *J. Virol.* **50**, 229–236.
Rosa, M. D., Gottlieb, E., Lerner, M. R. and Steitz, J. A. (1981). *Mol. Cell. Biol.* **1**, 785–796.
Rosen, H., Knoller, S. and Kaempfer, R. (1981). *Biochemistry* **20**, 3011–3020.
Rosenblum, M. G., Maxwell, B.L., Talpaz, M., Kelleher, P. J., McCredie, K. B. and Gutterman, J. U. (1986). *Cancer Res.* **46**, 4848–4852.
Rossi, G. B. (1985). *Interferon* **6**, 31–68.
Rozengurt, E., Rodriguez-Pena, M. and Smith, K. A. (1983). *Proc. Natl Acad. Sci. USA* **80**, 7244–7248.
Ryals, J., Dierks, P., Ragg, H. and Weissmann, C. (1985). *Cell* **41**, 497–507.

Sagar, A. D., Sehgal, P. B., Slate, D. L. and Ruddle, F. H. (1982). *J. Exp. Med.* **156**, 744–755.

Sagar, A. D., Sehgal, P. B., May, L. T., Inouye, M., Slate, D. L., Shulman, L. and Ruddle, F. H. (1984). *Science* **223**, 1312–1315.

Saiki, O. and Ralph, P. (1982). *Eur. J. Immunol.* **13**, 31–44.

Saltiel, A. R. and Cuatrecasas, P. (1986). *Proc. Natl Acad. Sci. USA* **83**, 5793–5797.

Saltiel, A. R., Fox, J. A., Sherline, P. and Cuatrecasas, P. (1986). *Science* **233**, 967–972.

Saltiel, A. R., Sherline, P. and Fox, J. A. (1987). *J. Biol. Chem.* **262,**1116–1121.

Samanta, H., Engel, D. A., Chao, H. M., Thakur, A., Garcia-Blanco, M. A. and Lengyel, P. (1986). *J. Biol. Chem.* **261**, 11849–11858.

Samid, D., Chang, E. H. and Friedman, R. M. (1984). *Biochem. Biophys. Res. Commun.* **119**, 21–28.

Samid, D., Chang, E. H. and Friedman, R. M. (1985). *Biochem. Biophys. Res. Commun.* **126**, 509–516.

Sanceau, J., Falcoff, R., Zilberstein, A., Beranger, F. and Vaquero, C. (1986). *J. Interferon Res.* **6**, Supplement 1, 55.

Scher, C. D., Dick, R. L., Whipple, A. P., Locatell, A. L. (1983). *Mol. Cell. Biol.* **3**, 70–81.

Schneck, J., Rager-Zisman, B., Rosen, O. M. and Bloom, B. R. (1982). *Proc. Natl Acad. Sci. USA* **79**, 1879–1883.

Schroder, E. W., Chou, I.-N., Jaken, S. and Black, P. H. (1978). *Nature (London)* **276**, 828–829.

Sehgal, P. B. (1982). *In* "Interferon 4" (I. Gresser, ed.), pp. 1–22. Academic Press.

Sehgal, P. B. and Sagar, A. D. (1980). *Nature (London)* **287**, 95–97.

Sehgal, P. B. and May, L. T. (1987). *J. Interferon Res.*, Supplement, in press.

Sehgal, P. B., Derman, E., Molloy, G. R., Tamm, I. and Darnell, J. E. (1976). *Science* **194**, 431–433.

Sehgal, P. B., Fraser, N. W. and Darnell, J. E. (1979). *Virology* **94**, 185–191.

Seghal, P. B., May, L. T., LaForge, K. S. and Inouye, M. (1982a). *Proc. Natl Acad. Sci. USA* **79**, 6932–6939.

Sehgal, P. B., Pfeffer, L. M. and Tamm, I. (1982b). *In* "Chemotherapy of Viral Infections" (P. E. Came and L. A. Caliguiri, eds), pp. 203–311. Springer-Verlag, Berlin.

Sehgal, P. B., Zilberstein, A., Ruggierrie, R. M., May, L. T., Ferguson-Smith, A., Slate, D. L. Revel, M. and Ruddle, F. H. (1986) *Proc. Natl Acad. Sci. USA* **83,** 5219–5222.

Sehgal, P. B., May, L. T., Tamm, I. and Vilček, J. (1987a). *Science* **235,** 731–732.

Sehgal, P. B., Walther, Z. and Tamm, I. (1987b). *Proc. Natl Acad. Sci. USA* **84,** 3663–3667.

Sergiescu, D., Gerfaux, J., Joret, A.-M. and Chany, C. (1986). *Proc. Natl Acad. Sci. USA* **83**, 5764–5768.

Shaw, A. R., Chan, J. K., Reid, S. and Seehafer, J. (1985). *JNCI* **6**, 1261–1268.

Shtivelman, E., Lifshitz, B., Gale, R. P. and Cananni, E. (1985). *Nature (London)* **315**, 550–554.

Slate, D. L. and Ruddle, F. H. (1979). *Cell* **16**, 171–180.

Smeland, E., Godal, T., Rund, E., Beiske, K. Funderud, S., Clark, E., Pfeifer-Ohlsson, S. and Ohlsson, R. (1985). *Proc. Natl Acad. Sci. USA* **82**, 6255–6259.

Smith, J. C. and Stiles, C. D. (1981). *Proc. Natl Acad. Sci. USA* **78**, 4363–4367.

Sokawa, Y., Watanabe, Y., Watanabe, Y. and Kawade, Y. (1977). *Nature (London)* **268**, 236–238.

Sokawa, Y., Nagata, K. and Ichikawa, Y. (1981). *Exp. Cell. Res.* **135**, 191–197.
Soslau, G., Bogucki, A. R., Gillespie, D. and Hubbell, H. R. (1984). *Biochem. Biophys. Res. Commun.* **119**, 941–948.
Spitzer, G., Verma, D. S., Beran, M., Zander, A. R., Dicke, K. A. and McCredie, K. B. (1981). *Blood* **57**, 71–74.
Spitzer, G., Verma, D. S., Beran, M., Zander, A. R., McCredie, K. B. and Dicke, K. A. (1982). *J. Natl Cancer Inst.* **68**, 35–42.
Sreevalsan, T., Rozengurt, E., Taylor-Papadimitriou, J. and Burchell, J. (1980). *J. Cell. Physiol.* **104**, 1–9.
St Laurent, G., Yoshie, O., Floyd-Smith, G., Samanta, H. and Sehgal, P. B. (1983). *Cell* **33**, 95–102.
Stadler, R., Müller, R. and Orfanos, C. E. (1986). *Br. J. Dermatol.* **114**, 723–277.
Staeheli, P., Haller, O., Boll, W., Lindenmann, J. and Weissman, C. (1986). *Cell* **44**, 147–158.
Stiles, C. D., Isberg, R. R., Pledger, W. J., Antoniades, H. N. and Scher, C. D. (1979). *J. Cell. Physiol.* **99**, 395–406.
Strayer, D. R., Weisband, J., Carter, W. A. and Brodsky, I. (1984). *In* "Human Tumor Cloning" (S. E. Salmon and J. M. Trent, eds), pp. 585–593. Grune and Stratton, New York.
Sugarman, B. J., Aggarwal, B. B., Hass, P. E., Figarri, I. S., Palladino, M. A. and Shepard, H. M. (1985). *Science* **230**, 943–945.
Sutherland, J., Mannoni, P., Rosa, F., Huyat, D., Turner, A. R. and Fellous, M. (1985). *Hum. Immunol.* **12**, 165–173.
Sutherland, J., Turner, A. R., Mannoni, P., McGann, L. E. and Turc, J. M. (1986). *J. Biol. Response Mod.* **5**, 250–262.
Talpaz, M., McCredie, K. B., Mavligit, G. M. and Gutterman, J. U. (1983). *Blood* **62**, 689–692.
Talpaz, M., Kantarjian, H. M., McCredie, K., Trujillo, J. M., Keating, M. J. and Gutterman, J. U. (1986). *New Eng. J. Med.* **314**, 1065–1069.
Tamm, I. (1977). *Proc. Natl Acad. Sci. USA* **74**, 5011–5015.
Tamm, I. and Kikuchi, T. (1979). *Proc. Natl Acad. Sci. USA* **76**, 5750–5754.
Tamm, I., Kikuchi, T., Darnell, J. E. Jr and Salditt-Georgieff, M. (1980). *Biochem.* **19**, 2743–2748.
Tamm, I., Pfeffer, L. M., Wang, E. and Murphy, J. S. (1984a). *Lymphokines* **9**, 37–70.
Tamm, I., Kikuchi, T., Wang, E. and Pfeffer, L. M. (1984b). *Cancer Res.* **44**, 2291–2296.
Tamm, I., Sehgal, P. B., Lamb, R. A. and Goldberg, A. R. (1984c). *In* "Antiviral Drugs and Interferon: The Molecular Basis of their Activity" (Y. Becker, ed.), pp. 203–252. Martinus Nijhoff, Boston.
Tamm, I., Jasny, B. R. and Pfeffer, L. M. (1987). *In* "Mechanisms of Interferon Actions" (L. M. Pfeffer, ed.) CRC Press, Inc. Boca Raton, FL. In press.
Taylor-Papadimitriou, J., Shearer, M. and Rozengurt, E. (1981). *J. Interferon Res.* **1**, 401–409.
Teranishi, T., Hirano, T., Arima, N. and Onoue, K. (1982). *J. Immunol.* **128**, 1903–1908.
Teranishi, T., Hirano, T., Lin, B.-H. and Onoue, K. (1984). *J. Immunol.* **133**, 3062–3067.
Thompson, M. R., Zhang, Z., Fournier, A. and Tan, Y. H. (1985). *J. Biol. Chem.* **260**, 563–567.
Tomida, Y. and Hasegawa, S. (1984). *Biochim. Biophys. Acta* **20**, 370–376.
Tominaga, S.-I. and Lengyel, P. (1985). *J. Biol. Chem.* **260**, 1975.

Torsteindottir, S., Masucci, M. G., Bejarano, M. T., Berthold, W., Klein, E. and Klein, G. (1985). *Cell Immunol.* **90**, 65–73.

Tovey, M. G. (1986). Results presented at the 1986 ISIR-TNO meeting on the Interferon System, Espoo, Finland, 7–12 September, 1986.

Tovey, M. G. and Gresser, I. (1985). *In* "The Biology of the Interferon System 1985" (W. E. Stewart II and H. Schellekens, eds), pp. 257–260. Elsevier Science Publishers B. V., Amsterdam.

Tovey, M. G., Dron, M., Mogenson, K. E., Lebleu, B., Mehti, N. and Begon-Lours-Guymarko, L. (1983). *J. Gen. Virol.* **64**, 2649–2653.

Traub, A., Feinstein, S., Gez, M., Lazar, A. and Mizrahi, A. (1984). *J. Biol. Chem.* **259**, 13872–13877.

Van Damme, J., Openakker, G., Simpson, R. J., Rubira, M. R., Cayphas, S., Vink, A., Billiau, A. and Van Snick, J. (1985). *J. Exp. Med.* **165,** 914–919.

Vandenbussche, P., Divizia, M., Verhaegen-Lewalle, M., Fuse, A., Kuwata, T., De Clerq, E. and Content, J. (1981). *Virol* **111**, 11–22.

Vaquero, C., Sanceau, J., Weissenbach, J., Beranger, F. and Falcoff, R. (1986). *J. Interferon Res.* **6**, 161–170.

Vasavada, R., Eager, K. B., Barbanti-Brodano, G., Caputo, A. and Ricciardi, R. P. (1986). *Proc. Natl Acad. Sci. USA* **83**, 5257–5261.

Verhagen-Lewalle, M., Divizia, M., Vandenbussche, P., Kuwata, T. and Content, J. (1980). *Proc. Natl Acad. Sci. USA* **77**, 4479–4483.

Verhagen-Lewalle, M., Kuwata, T., Zhang, Z.-X., De Clercq, E., Cantell, K. and Content, J. (1982). *Virol.* **117**, 425–434.

Verma, D. S., Spitzer, G., Gutterman, J. U., Zander, A. R., McCredie, K. B. and Dicke, K. A. (1979). *Blood* **54**, 1423–1427.

Vilček, J. (1987). *In* "Frontiers in Microbiology" (A. Billiau, ed.). In press.

Vilček, J., Palombella, V. J., Henrikson-DeStefano, D., Swenson, C., Feinman, R., Hirai, M. and Tsujimoto, M. (1986). *J. Exp. Med.* **163**, 632–643.

Vogel, J., Kress, M., Khoury, G. and Gilbert, J. (1986). *Mol. Cell. Biol.* **6**, 3550–3554.

Wallach, D., Fellous, M. and Revel, M. (1982). *Nature (London)* **299**, 833–836.

Walther, Z., May, L. T. and Sehgal, P. B. (1987). In preparation.

Wang, E., Pfeffer, L. M. and Tamm, I. (1981). *Proc. Natl Acad. Sci. USA* **78**, 6281–6285.

Wang, E., Michl, J., Pfeffer, L. M., Silverstein, S. C. and Tamm, I. (1984). *J. Cell Biol.* **98**, 1328–1341.

Weissenbach, J., Chernajorsky, Y., Zeevi, M., Shulman, L., Soreq, H., Nir, U., Dallach, D., Perricaudet, M., Trollais, P. and Revel, M. (1980). *Proc. Natl Acad. Sci. USA* **77**, 7152–7156.

Wells, J. A. Swyryd, E. A. and Stark, G. R. (1984). *J. Biol. Chem.* **259**, 1363–1370.

Wells, V. and Mallucci, L. (1985). *Exp. Cell. Res.* **159**, 27–36.

Weinberg, R. A. (1985). *Science* **230**, 770–776.

Whitaker-Dowling, P. A. and Younger, J. S. (1983). *Virology* **131**, 128–136.

Whitaker-Dowling, P. A. and Younger, J. S. (1984). *Virology* **137**, 171–181.

Whitaker-Dowling, P. A., Wilcox, D. K., Widnell, C. C. and Younger, J. S. (1983). *Proc. Natl Acad. Sci. USA* **80**, 1083–1086.

Wilcox, D. K., Whitaker-Dowling, P. A. Younger, J. S. and Widnell, C. C. (1983). *Mol. Cell. Biol.* **3**, 1533–1536.

Wong, G. H. W. and Goeddel, D. V. (1986). *Nature (London)* **323**, 819–822.

Yaar, M., Karassik, R. L., Schnipper, L. E. and Gilchrest, B. A. (1985). *J. Invest. Dermatol.* **1**, 70–74.

Yaar, M., Palleroni, A. V. and Gilchrest, B. A. (1986). *J. Cell Biol.* **103**, 1349–1354.

Yang, K., Samanta, H., Dougherty, J., Bettadapura, J., Broeze, R. and Lengyel, P. (1981). *J. Biol. Chem.* **256**, 9324–9328.

Yap, W. H., Teo, T. S. and Tan, Y. H. (1986a). *Science* **234**, 355–358.

Yap, W. H., Teo, T. S., McCoy, E. and Tan, Y. H. (1986b). *Proc. Natl Acad. Sci. USA* **83**, 7765–7769.

Yarden, A., Shure-Gottlieb, H., Chebath, J., Revel, M. and Kimchi, A. (1984). *EMBO J.* **3**, 969–973.

Zilberstein, A., Ruggieri, R., Korn, J. H. and Revel, M. (1986). *EMBO J.* **5**, 2529–2437.

Zinkernagel, R. M. and Doherty, P. C. (1979). *Adv. Immunol.* **27**, 51–177.

Zinn, K. and Maniatis, T. (1986). *Cell* **45**, 611–618.

Zoon, K. C., Arnheiter, H., Zur Nedden, D. L., FitzGerald, D. J. P. and Willingham, M. G. (1983). *Virology* **130**, 195–203.

Zoon, K. C., Karasaki, Y., Zur Nedden, D. L., Hu, R. and Arnheiter, H. (1986a). *Proc. Natl Acad. Sci. USA* **83**, 8226–8230.

Zoon, K. C., Arnheiter, H., Zur Nedden, D. L., FitzGerald, D. J. P. and Willingham, M. G. (1986b). *Virology* **130**, 195–203.

Zullo, J. N., Cochran, B. H., Huang, A. S. and Stiles, C. D. (1985). *Cell* **43**, 793–800.

NOTE ADDED IN PROOF

Human IFN-β_2 has now also been recognized to be identical to the monocyte-derived hepatocyte-stimulating factor (HSF) (J. Gauldie, C. Richards, D. Harnish, P. Lansdorp and H. Baumann, *Proc. Natl Acad. Sci. USA,* submitted). Human monocytes exposed to stimuli such as the *E. coli* endotoxin or lipopolysaccharide (LPS) secrete HSF which is involved in eliciting the "acute phase response" in the liver, characterized by decreased synthesis of albumin and increased synthesis of fibrinogen, haptoglobin, α_2-macroglobulin and C-reactive protein (reviewed in I. Kushner, J. E. Volanakis, H. Gewurz, *NY Acad. Sci.* **389,** 1–479, 1982).

LPS derived from strains of *E. coli* and *S. typhimurium* rapidly elevate IFN-β_2, but not IFN-β_1, mRNA levels in human fibroblasts (FS-4 strain) (D. C. Helfgott, L. T. May, Z. Sthoeger, I. Tamm and P. B. Sehgal, *Science,* submitted). Cultures of LPS-treated FS-4 cells exhibit an antiviral state against vesicular stomatitis virus which can be prevented by anti-IFN-β antiserum. Medium from LPS-treated FS-4 cell cultures enhances the number of immunoglobulin-secreting cells in cultures of human B-lymphoblastoid (CESS) cells. Thus, in the course of infection due to Gram-negative bacteria, LPS may trigger host defence mechanisms not only be enhancement of B-cell proliferation and monocyte/macrophage activation, but also by its enhancement of IFN-β_2 secretion by the ubiquitous fibroblast.

It has been reported that preparations of IFN-β_2 produced by *Xenopus laevis* oocytes microinjected with synthetic chimeric IFN-β_2 mRNA do not possess detectable antiviral activity when assayed on human cells although they support the growth of certain murine plasmacytoma cells and produce a two-fold increase in immunoglobulin secretion by human CESS cells (P. Poupart, P. Vandenabeele, S. Cayphas, J. Van Snick, G. Haegeman, V. Kruys, W. Fiers and J. Content, *EMBO J.* **6,** 1219–1224, 1987). These investigators view their observations as in conflict with those of Zilberstein *et al.* (1986) who expressed IFN-β_2 cDNA and genomic DNA clones in a variety of mammalian expression systems to yield IFN-β_2 preparations with clear antiviral activity on human but not on murine cells. We do not view these two reports as incompatible, as the possibility is left open that additional post-transcriptional events may have occurred in the mammalian expression systems used by Zilberstein *et al.* (1986), which did not take place in the system used by Poupart *et al.* (1987). It has been observed previously that IFN-β (presumably IFN-β_1) when synthesized and processed in a number of different heterologous translation systems does not display antiviral activity (P. B. Sehgal, B. Dobberstein and I. Tamm, *Proc. Natl Acad. Sci. USA* **74,** 3409–3414, 1977).

Fujita *et al.* (T. Fujita, H. Shibuya, H. Hotta, K. Yamanishi & T. Taniguchi, *Cell* **49,** 357–367, 1987) could not identify any negative regulatory sequence element(s) within the IFN-β_1 promoter that need to be derepressed during induction. However, Fujita *et al.* (1987) showed that induction of IFN-β_1 is regulated by repeated sequence units each consisting of 6 base pairs (AAGTGA is the most efficient) in a manner consistent with a "positive enhancer" model of induction.

Interferons and Autoimmunity

MARC FELDMANN, MARCO LONDEI AND GLENN BUCHAN

Charing Cross Sunley Research Centre, Lurgan Avenue, Hammersmith, London, W6 8LW.

I INTRODUCTION

In the past few years data has accumulated that the tissue cells in the majority of human autoimmune diseases express abnormally elevated levels of HLA class II antigens, for example in thyroiditis, diabetes and rheumatoid arthritis (Table I). Similar overexpression has been found in murine autoimmune

INTERFERON 9
ISBN 0 12 302558 3

TABLE I Autoimmune Diseases

With excess class II on target
Graves', Hashimoto's, Insulin dependent diabetes, rheumatoid arthritis, Sjogren's, biliary cirrhosis, coeliac, multiple sclerosis.
Without excess class II on target
Myasthenia gravis
? Haemopoietic (unassessable)

diseases (e.g. MRL/1pr mice, Kelley and Roths, 1982). Because the expression of HLA class II is essential (but not necessarily sufficient) for the activation of T helper cells, these observations were instrumental in the generation of the concept that autoimmunity is perpetuated (and conceivably also initiated) by the antigen-presenting capacity of the target tissues, for example the thyroid epithelial cells (thyrocytes) in Graves' hyperthyroidism (Bottazzo *et al.*, 1983).

There is evidence that all interferons (IFNs) (α, β, γ) are inducers of HLA class I (HLA-A, -B or -C) but the bulk of the evidence suggests that only IFN-γ induces class II, with the exception that *in vivo* treatment with IFN-α causes augmented monocyte class II expression (Rhodes *et al.*, 1983).

These results have led to an examination of the role of IFNs, especially IFN-γ, in autoimmunity, at both the conceptual and experimental level. This review will attempt to summarize our understanding of the published data and our unpublished data in October 1986. For a broader view of the involvement of interferons in disease, see Gresser (1982).

II AN OVERALL CONCEPT OF AUTOIMMUNITY

The first formulation of the "class II overexpression" concept of autoimmunity was published in 1983 in collaboration with Franco Bottazzo's group, with particular reference to endocrine autoimmunity (Bottazzo *et al.*, 1983). We currently think that, with minor modifications, this concept provides an overall framework for understanding the chronic phase of autoimmunity, including that found in non-endocrine diseases, such as rheumatoid arthritis and Sjogren's syndrome. The latest version is described by Feldmann *et al.* (1987). The role of genetic predisposition and environmental agents will be discussed subsequently.

Figure 1 illustrates this concept and highlights the importance of the molecules inducing class II expression, as these control a predictable chain of activation events ending in inflammation and tissue damage.

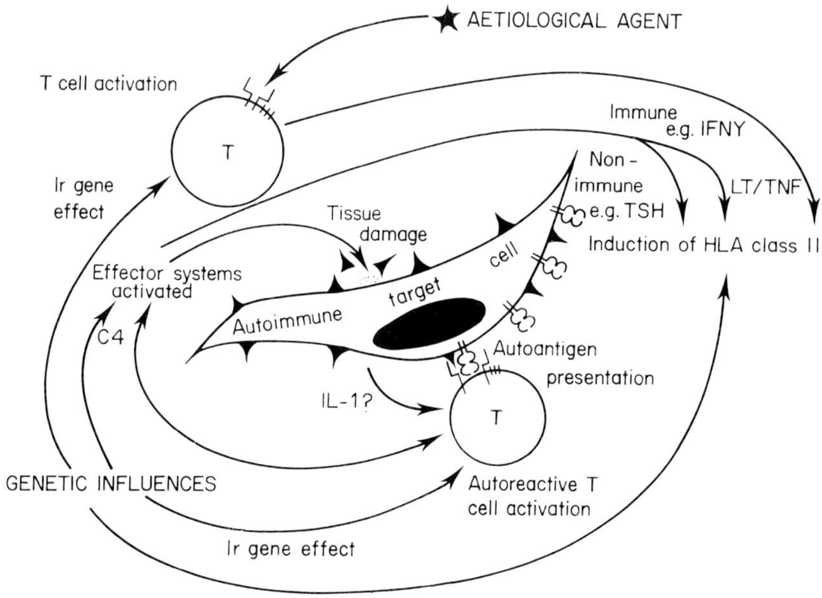

Fig. 1 Vicious cycle of autoimmunity: a pictorial representation of multifactorial influences determining whether an autoimmune response becomes chronic or resolves.

The key predictions of this model have been tested using thyroid disease as a model. Thus it was found that products of activated T cells can induce class II (Todd *et al.*, 1985). Such class II-expressing thyrocytes could present antigen to T cell clones (Londei *et al.*, 1984). Most importantly, thyroid tissue in Graves' thyroiditis (a typical autoimmune disease characterized by the presence of an autoantibody, termed long-acting thyroid stimulator, which acts as an agonist of the receptor for thyroid stimulating hormone (TSH)) contains activated T lymphocytes which are stimulated by autologous thyrocytes, but not by autologous blood cells (Londei *et al.*, 1985). The implications of these three types of experiments and subsequent investigations in these areas are discussed below.

III REGULATION OF HLA CLASS II EXPRESSION

In the absence of disease, dendritic cells, Langerhans cells, thymus epithelial cells, B cells, activated T cells, and monocytes, express class II. Epithelia, such as on large bronchi and gut, usually express in some areas. Whether this should be considered "normal" or due to environmental insult is unclear.

Lactating breast epithelium expresses class II, suggesting the possibility of hormonal regulation (Klareskog *et al.*, 1980).

The expression of HLA class II antigens (HLA-DR, -DP and -DQ in humans) on various cell types may be classified into broad groups.

(a) Constitutive. Dendritic cells, B lymphocytes and thymic epithelial cells express at high levels in the absence of obvious extraneous inducers, and maintain expression when put in tissue culture, so this is termed "constitutive expression", although this does not imply that it cannot be augmented (as B cells augment surface class II in response to LPS, BSFp1 or IL-4, anti-Ig).

(b) Inducible. This group includes many and perhaps most cell types. Normally, blood monocytes express class II, but this diminishes rapidly in culture in the absence of stimulation by IFN-γ. Fibroblasts and endothelial cells are inducible by IFN-γ (Collins *et al.*, 1984), as are thyrocytes. Activated human T lymphocytes express HLA class II.

(c) Non-expressing. Whether any cell type is totally unable to express class II is not clear. Cells very early in the B cell lineage or very late, e.g. plasma cells, do not express class II. So far oligodendrocytes have not been demonstrated to express class II *in vivo* or *in vitro*, but possibly this reflects the fact that the appropriate inducers have not been elucidated. In principle there is no reason why any cell could not be induced, and a simplifying notion is that under appropriate circumstances all cells may be able to act as antigen-presenting cells, at least for antigens already present on their surface, or small peptides.

In analysing the induction of class II on thyrocytes it was found that IFN-γ induced class II expression, of all three types HLA-DR, -DP and -DQ, although with a gradient of efficiency, i.e. DR > DP > DQ at all concentrations of IFN-γ, with DQ expression requiring the highest concentration of IFN-γ (Todd *et al.*, 1987a). Natural or recombinant IFN-α and -β or IL-2 did not induce class II. Subsequent analysis has revealed that TSH synergizes with IFN-γ, but it is not clear whether it has any effect by itself (Todd *et al.*, 1987b), especially in view of reports that there are circulating IFN-γ-releasing cells, detected by a reversed plaque forming assay (Martinez-Maza *et al.*, 1984).

The synergistic effect of TSH on thyroid class II expression suggests that the target tissue of an autoimmune disease can contribute to its maintenance. The levels of TSH required to synergize with IFN-γ can be found in Hashimoto's thyroiditis (0.1 mU/ml). In contrast, in Graves' disease TSH levels are very low, but the TSH agonist antibody "long acting thyroid stimulator" (LATS) could mimic the TSH effects.

Islet cells of the pancreas are the target cells of juvenile, insulin-dependent (or type I) diabetes mellitus (IDDM). During the disease process, access to tissue is very difficult to obtain, but in the rare event of death in the early stages of the disease, it has been demonstrated that the remaining insulin-producing B cells express HLA class II (Bottazzo *et al.*, 1985; Foulis and Farquarson, 1986). This suggests that IDDM fits into the same pattern of disease as proposed, and so it is a question of interest to determine the nature of the HLA class II inducers active on human islet cells. Pujol-Borrell *et al.* (1986) found that neither IFN-γ, -α, -β, nor about 12 other ligands were able to induce HLA class II expression. In contrast it has recently been found that high concentrations of IFN-γ induce low levels of class II expression in mouse islet cells (Wright *et al.*, 1986). More recently we have found that IFN-γ, in synergy with either TNF or LT, strongly induced class II expression in islet cells (Pujol-Borrell *et al.*, 1987). This observation suggests that synergy of mediators may be an important principle in the precise regulation of HLA class II expression, with different cell types responding to different ligands.

A summary of known current inducers of HLA class II is shown in Table I, which we are sure is incomplete.

TABLE II Summary of Induction of HLA class II

Cell type	Inducer
Monocyte	IFN-γ and LT or TNF
Fibroblast	IFN-γ
Endothelium	IFN-γ
Thyrocyte	IFN-γ and TSH
Astrocyte	IFN-γ
β islet cell	IFN-γ and LT or TNF
Oligodendrocyte	IFN-γ and ?
B cell	Crosslinked Ig, IL-4, LPS, ?IFN-γ
T cell	Crosslinked TR, ?IL-2 and IFN-γ

Abbreviations: IFN-γ, interferon-γ; TSH, thyroid stimulating hormone; LT, lymphotoxin; TNF, tumour necrosis factor; Ig, immunoglobulin; IL-4, interleukin-4, formerly BSF-1, B cell stimulating factor 1; LPS, lipopolysaccharide; TR, T cell receptor for antigen; IL-2, interleukin-2.

IV ABILITY OF THYROID EPITHELIUM TO ACT AS ANTIGEN-PRESENTING CELLS

Expression of HLA class II by thyrocytes and other targets of autoimmune diseases has usually been assessed by fluorescence microscopy using monoclonal antibodies. This does not establish that these cells synthesized the class II antigens detected, as it is possible (but not likely) that these were picked up from infiltrating lymphoid cells. Thus it was important to establish that purified thyrocytes were capable of presenting antigen in functional tests. This has been done in several ways, using influenza peptide-specific T cell clones (Londei *et al.*, 1984), or thyrocyte-specific autoreactive clones (Londei *et al.*, 1985). A problem of these experiments is how to be sure that it is thyrocytes themselves presenting antigen, and not the few residual macrophages or dendritic cells. In the case of influenza virus responses, this was resolved by observations that thyrocytes could not present whole influenza virus, but only peptides, i.e. they could not process antigen effectively. This result reconciles possibly conflicting concepts, e.g. if any cell which can be induced to express HLA class II can act as an antigen-presenting cell, why has there been an evolution of specialized antigen-presenting cells: macrophages, dendritic cells, Langerhans cells etc? From the incapacity of thyrocytes to process an infectious agent (influenza virus), it seems clear that the specialized antigen-presenting cells are essential for large antigens such as viruses and bacteria, but the antigen-presenting function of epithelia would be sufficient to render surface autoantigens immunogenic in the presence of class II expression.

With thyroid-specific T cell lines, it has been easy to exclude presentation by non-thyrocytes: these do not activate, presumably as they lack the thyrocyte-specific antigens (Grubeck-Loebenstein, Londei and Feldmann, unpublished observations).

V THYROCYTE-SPECIFIC CLONES INFILTRATE THE TARGET TISSUE DURING AN AUTOIMMUNE DISEASE

This concept of autoimmunity has been successfully and extensively tested in Graves' disease, because this is the autoimmune thyroid disease most commonly operated on. Almost 20 patients have been investigated, and all have thyrocyte-specific T cells infiltrating the gland. These have been cloned from six individuals by stimulation with mitogen-free IL-2, and the pattern of clones derived was reproducible: $\sim 10\%$ of thyroid-specific clones; $\sim 5\%$ of autologous MLR clones; $\sim 80\%$ of clones of unknown specificity. However, there are still a number of gaps in our knowledge of the steps occurring in this hypothetical scheme of the mechanism of autoimmunity, e.g. (i) Do the target cells synthesize HLA class II? (ii) Where does the IL-1 needed for T cell activation come from? Can epithelial cells make IL-1 (iii) Is there sufficient IFN-γ present in autoimmune disease tissue, such as in Graves' disease, to mediate the HLA class II expression detected, and necessary for antigen-presenting function?

These questions are currently being addressed in two ways: first, by examining tissue biopsy samples and analysing them for mRNA content (for IFN-γ and other genes), and also by cloning T cells infiltrating the autoimmune tissue and determining their capacity to produce IFN-γ. These approaches will be discussed separately.

VI LYMPHOKINE PRODUCTION BY AUTOREACTIVE CLONES

Recently we have been interested in applying the T cell cloning approach to the events taking place locally during the autoimmune process. Thus we have been cloning cells from autoimmune hypothyroidism (Hashimoto's thyroiditis), and rheumatoid arthritis, using protocols based on those initially described using Graves' disease.

Currently our protocol involves an initial selection in recombinant IL-2, and the cells are also stimulated with anti-CD3 antibody and autologous APC at a stage where only the cells activated *in vivo* remain. Anti-CD3 was chosen as the nonspecific stimulus because the antibody binds to a molecular cluster adjacent to the T cell receptor for antigen, and so this should closely mimic stimulation by antigen and antigen-presenting cells (Londei *et al.*, 1987).

With this procedure we have obtained clones of T cells from Hashimoto's thyroiditis and rheumatoid arthritis. These have been characterized for the production of lymphokines, including IFN-γ. This was assayed by a commercial radioimmunoassay (Boots-Celltech). Because it seems clear from our previous work that IFN-γ is important in the pathogenesis of Hashimoto's thyroiditis, it was of interest that rheumatoid arthritis clones produced significantly more IFN-γ than those derived from Hashimoto's thyroiditis. This difference may have been due to different cell phenotypes, as it is widely believed that $CD4^+$ cells produce more lymphokines than $CD8^+$ cells. Thus lymphokine production, especially of IFN-γ, was correlated to CD4 or $CD8^+$ phenotype in clones derived from Hashimoto's thyroiditis, where CD8 clones predominate. The results, on a small number of clones, were clear-cut. There was no diminution in IFN-γ production by CD8 clones (in fact, it averaged higher than CD4 clones), and so the lesser IFN-γ production of Hashimoto's thyroiditis compared to rheumatoid arthritis was not due to different CD4/CD8 phenotypes. However, comparison of clones from only two patients does not permit any generalization.

It was of interest to investigate whether other lymphokines which synergize with IFN-γ were also produced by the same infiltrating T cell clones derived from autoimmune sites. Tumour necrosis factor and lymphotoxin, two closely related molecules which synergize with IFN-γ in a number of ways (e.g. in cytotoxicity, activation of macrophage antiviral effect, induction of class II), were also produced by some of these clones (unpublished data).

VII EXPRESSION OF LYMPHOKINE AND CYTOKINE mRNA IN AUTOIMMUNE TISSUE BIOPSIES

The problems of assaying lymphokine production from diseased tissue are well known. Sensitivity and complexity of bioassays can be a problem, and adsorption, consumption, lability and enzymatic degradation add to the problems caused by potential inhibitors and antagonists. Some of these problems can be overcome by the use of binding assays such as radioimmunoassays or enzyme-linked immunoassays, but only a few as yet have the desired sensitivity, e.g. IFN-γ radioimmunoassays.

With the cloning of important mediator molecules, such as IFNs, it is possible to use gene probes to analyse the expression of mRNA for mediator molecules in autoimmune disease tissues, provided local biopsy material is available. We have thus been assaying synovial fluid and membrane samples of patients with rheumatoid arthritis, and have found that such an analysis is not only possible but highly informative, and has an important advantage of universality, the same technique being used for all assays, with only the cDNA probe differing, and of sensitivity, with 2×10^6 cells sufficing for 8–10 probings.

With these techniques, it has been possible to evaluate whether IFN-γ mRNA is present in autoimmune disease tissues. The results in rheumatoid arthritis are quite clear: mRNA for IFN-γ is present. The levels of mRNA are quite low if compared to optimally stimulated peripheral blood lymphoid cells (Buchan *et al.*, in preparation).

The kinetics of IFN-γ mRNA stability can be investigated by placing cells in culture, without any other stimulus. This revealed that the levels of mRNA were virtually unchanged for 3–5 days of culture. The kinetics of IFN-γ mRNA after stimulation of PBL with a mitogen mixture (phytohaemagglutinin and phorbol dibutyrate) showed a rapid onset with a peak at 4–8 hours, and return to low levels by 24 hours. These low levels were still expressed at 48 hours, suggesting that in rheumatoid arthritis joint cells we may be observing activated T cells. Two out of eight patients studied showed high levels of IFN-γ mRNA expression throughout a 5-day period, suggesting that there may be a self-perpetuating system of cellular–molecular interactions which maintains the rate of IFN-γ synthesis.

Thyroid autoimmune tissues have not been as extensively investigated as rheumatoid arthritis, but IFN-γ mRNA has been found in Graves' disease (Buchan *et al.*, unpublished data).

Regrettably, it is not easy to estimate IFN protein levels from mRNA levels, and so we do not know whether these are high or low. However, there is evidence that in certain cell types, e.g. human fibroblasts, or the THP-1 monocytic cell line, HLA class II induction may occur at 0.1 U/ml of IFN-γ or less (G. Portillo *et al.*, unpublished data), and so it seems likely that there is sufficient IFN-γ mRNA to induce class II expression. This is especially the case as there are other molecules which could synergize with IFN-γ for class II expression, e.g. TNF (Pujol-Borrell *et al.*, 1987), which we have also shown to be present in autoimmune tissues, in the rheumatoid joint (Buchan *et al.*, 1987).

Other workers have used antibodies to stain cells containing IFN and so presumably producing it. This technique is not easy, but it has been reported that IFN-α and -γ are present in dermatomyositis (Isenberg *et al.*, 1986), but only IFN-γ in Sjogren's syndrome (Rowe, Isenberg *et al.*, unpublished data).

VIII HLA CLASS II mRNA ANALYSES OF THYROID AUTOIMMUNE TISSUES

It is implicit in our formulation of autoimmunity that the target tissue synthesizes HLA class II, and thus becomes capable of presenting its own autoantigens. The capacity of thyrocytes to synthesize HLA class II has been investigated using cDNA probes to class II antigens (DR, DP and DQ) and the results can be summarized:

(a) Thyrocytes extracted and purified from Graves' disease tissue synthesize as much DRα mRNA as the lymphoid and monocyte cells infiltrating the tissues. Thus even while it is impossible to obtain pure populations of thyrocytes, it is evident that thyrocytes are synthesizing DRα in Graves' thyroiditis.

(b) Thyrocytes purified from non-autoimmune states (e.g. nodular goitre) can be induced by IFN-γ to produce DRα, DPα and DQ$\alpha\alpha$ mRNA.

Taken together the above observations indicate that the class II antigens detected on the surfaces of thyrocytes were synthesized by them. Further evidence is that thyrocyte mRNA induced by IFN-γ for DRα is enhanced by thyroid stimulating hormone (Londei *et al.*, 1987a).

IX IL-1 mRNA IN AUTOIMMUNE TISSUES

Induction of many immune responses requires the presence of IL-1. It was thus of interest to determine whether there is IL-1 present in autoimmune tissues, and more specifically whether IL-1 is synthesized by the target tissue, thyrocytes. We have initiated studies of this type, which are limited by the difficulties in separating thyrocytes (highly adherent) from monocytes/macrophages. Preliminary results indicate that there is abundant IL-1 in Graves' disease tissue; fractionation into the thyrocyte-enriched and mononuclear fractions revealed that both contained abundant IL-1 mRNA. As the thyrocyte-enriched fraction has far fewer macrophages than the mononuclear fraction, it seems likely that the thyrocytes can produce IL-1 and this could be important in the early stages of the disease (unpublished data). In the later stages of the disease, there is an abundant lymphocyte and monocyte infiltrate, which could contribute IL-1.

In rheumatoid arthritis, we have performed more extensive studies (Buchan *et al.*, 1987, submitted for publication), and it is evident that all biopsy samples of active rheumatoid arthritis, either of digested synovial membrane or synovial fluid cells, contain mRNA for IL-1, both α and β. It was of interest that in optimally activated PBL the IL-1α/β ratio is about 1:3, whereas the ratio of α/β in the rheumatoid arthritis joints was about 1:1. Currently there is little information available about stimuli inducing IL-1α or β differentially, or different cell types producing IL-1α or β selectively.

X DOES INTERFERON THERAPY IN HUMANS CAUSE AUTOIMMUNITY?

From the discussions above, it might be anticipated that IFN therapy, as in IFN trials, could induce autoimmunity. However, it is known that the half-life of systemically administered IFN is very short, and so it is not clear how much would reach potential sites of autoimmunity. Nor is it known how the many effects of IFN would balance out—class II expression obviously favours autoimmunity, but other effects, e.g. anti-proliferative effects, could restore the balance.

It was of interest that the IFN-α trials have produced a variety of reports of autoimmunity. One by Fentiman *et al.* (1985) reported that 3/7 patients with breast cancer given Namalwa IFN-α (a mixture of about eight types) for up to 1 year developed hypothyroidism. Burman *et al.* (1985) reported that in patients with carcinoid tumour 6/41 developed thyroid dysfunction, 4 being hypothyroidism and 2 hyperthyroidism. Five out of 6 of these developed classical thyroid autoantibodies in their serum, as did 5 other patients who did not develop a clinical disease. Other cases have been found in IFN trials but not published as yet (personal communication).

The results available to us so far are from IFN-α trials, which were initiated earlier than the IFN-γ trials. The effects of IFN-α on class II expression are not as well documented as those of IFN-γ. Monocyte class II expression of recipients during Namalwa IFN-α trials has been reported, but *in vitro* IFN-α does not induce class II expression, apart from a report with IFN-α_2 (Rhodes *et al.*, 1985).

It is possible that, *in vivo*, IFN-α initiates a pathway which ends up inducing IFN-γ, possibly in LGL cells. These are known to be activated by IFN-α, and are capable of producing IFN-γ.

A question of interest is whether sufficient IFN-γ is generated following viral infections to be available to induce class II. With the development of a radioimmunoassay for IFN-γ, it has become possible to investigate this, and it has been reported that in CSF of individuals with viral meningitis there is abundant IFN-γ (Abbott *et al.*, 1985), on average 5 U/ml, sufficient to induce class II on many tissues.

Thus it appears that the induction of class II *in vivo* as a consequence of IFN-γ production during an infectious episode is entirely plausible.

XI GENETIC SUSCEPTIBILITY, IFNs AND AUTOIMMUNITY

A number of experiments suggest that the response of individuals (animals or humans) to IFNs may depend on various genes. In the context of autoimmunity, a number of recent observations suggest that perhaps genotype may contribute to variations in the response to IFNs, and perhaps subsequent predisposition to autoimmunity.

(a) Fontana *et al.* (personal communication) have reported that SJL astrocytes (a strain sensitive to experimental allergic encephalitis) respond to IFN-γ at lower doses than BALB/c astrocytes (a resistant mouse strain).

(b) Massa *et al.* (1986) have demonstrated that JHM virus can induce class II expression in cultured astrocytes. This occurs more readily in mouse strains susceptible to demyelination induced by this virus (V. ter Meulen, personal communication).

(c) Rat strains differ in their expression of class II antigens in islets of pancreas (Ulrichs *et al.*, 1986). Islet cells of BB/W rats, prone to insulin-dependent diabetes mellitus, can be induced to express class II by IFN whereas those of non-diabetic strains cannot (Walker *et al.*, 1986). This observation may be due to prior exposure *in vivo* to activating agents such as TMF.

(d) Guinea pigs of the $(2 \times 13)F_1$ strain during EAE show much greater expression of the class II antigens of the allele susceptible to the disease, as detected in brain sections of affected animals (Sobel and Colwin, 1986).

It is not clear whether these recent observations, none as yet fully documented, represent a genetic susceptibility to respond differently to IFNs or other agents. Analogous studies in humans are not easy to perform, due to limited availability of tissues, but it is conceivable that tissues of individuals with autoimmunity may respond differently from tissues of those without. We are attempting to test this with thyroid tissue, but even if differences were to be found, it would not be easy to establish that the human results were part of a genetic predisposition.

Of the human autoimmune diseases, a large cluster are associated with a higher relative risk in DR3 individuals. These include insulin-dependent diabetes mellitus, Sjogren's syndrome, SLE and Graves' disease, primary biliary cirrhosis, myasthenia gravis, Addison's disease (see Immunological Reviews, Vol. 70).

Initially, there appear to be "too many" DR3-associated diseases, suggesting perhaps a common diathesis rather than a specific response to any single agent. This has led us to perform a number of pilot studies. One was to ask whether the PBL of DR3 individuals make more IFN-γ in response to a mitogenic stimulus. No differences were found (Londei, M., Feldmann, M. and Balkwill, F., unpublished data). Another was to try and determine whether $DR3^+$ thyroids respond to IFN-γ more strongly than $DR3^-$ thyroids. No difference has been noted so far (Todd *et al.*, unpublished data).

However, differential responses to IFN-γ or IFN-γ and another lymphokine or cytokine, e.g. TNF, cannot be excluded as a factor in the aetiology of human autoimmune diseases.

The synergy of TNF or LT with IFN-γ in a variety of phenomena—cytotoxicity, class II induction, IL-1 induction, antiviral effect—may be of importance in autoimmunity. In this context, it is of interest that TNF and LT genes map within HLA in humans (Spies *et al.,* 1986) and in H2 in mice.

XII CLASS I REGULATION BY IFNs: ROLE IN AUTOIMMUNITY

Much discussion, in this article and previously, has highlighted the role of IFNs in regulating class II. However, IFN-α, -β and -γ all regulate class I antigens and it is apparent from immunohistological studies that class I expression is also abnormal in autoimmune diseases such as thyroiditis and diabetes.

Enhanced class I expression would be of importance in permitting class I restricted cytotoxic T cells to recognize their target more effectively. There is evidence that the density of class I expression is highly relevant to the capacity of CTL to kill their targets, in virally infected cells.

IFNs are not the only molecules which regulate class I antigens—TNF by itself induces class I gene expression (Collins *et al.,* 1984), and we have found TNF to be present in the autoimmune tissues of rheumatoid arthritis.

XIII DOES THE MECHANISM OF INITIATION OF AUTOIMMUNITY DIFFER FROM THAT OF MAINTENANCE?

Most of the data that can be assembled in human diseases refers to the established disease, and so refers to the maintenance phase of the disease. It is not known whether the initiation phase is necessarily identical.

Our own preference is that the earliest event in autoimmunity is viral infection, leading to the production of IFNs and other lymphokines, especially TNF and LT. The antigen-presenting cells of importance in this response would be "professional" antigen-presenting cells such as macrophages or dendritic cells, as we have obtained evidence (Londei *et al.*, 1984) that tissue cells such as thyrocytes cannot present intact viruses to T helper cells due to lack of "processing" capacity.

However, once T cell activation yielding IFN-γ and other signals occurs and class II expression on the target tissue is induced, the activation of autoreactive T cells takes place, and from this time on the lymphokine generation by the autoreactive T cells is of importance in maintaining the autoreactive process.

It is a point of interest as to why organ-specific autoreactive precursors are present, capable of being activated if the tissues express class II. We have discussed this at length elsewhere (Feldmann *et al.*, 1985, 1986, 1987). It is pertinent that if nude mice are grafted with a rat thymus, permitting T cell development to occur in the adult phase, the animals have organ-specific antibodies typical of the human organ-specific autoimmune diseases (Taguchi *et al.*, 1986). Thus a deeper understanding of the process of T cell tolerance is vital for understanding the process of autoimmunization. Our own view is that efficient "non-responsiveness" to self, regardless of the mechanism (e.g. clonal deletion, clonal "anergy", suppressor T cells), effectively causes a "hole in the repertoire", a shape that cannot be recognized by T cells. If there are too many holes in the repertoire, the capacity to recognize foreign antigens becomes progressively more restricted. Hence there must be a balance between the efficiency of self-unresponsiveness and of response to extrinsic agents. For antigens only present on rare target cells, lacking in class II, it would be difficult to engage any of the known mechanisms of non-responsiveness, and this may account for the predisposition to organ-specific autoimmunity, as the precursor cells are present; capable of being activated.

XIV ROLE OF ATYPICAL IFNs IN AUTOIMMUNITY

An unusual type of IFN, acid-labile IFN-α, has been found in the serum of patients with SLE, scleroderma, Sjogren's and occasionally rheumatoid arthritis, with a higher incidence in those with active SLE. Not all patients, usually 50% or less, have elevated titres (usually in the range 8–32, Preble *et al.* (1982)). A similar type of acid-labile IFN has been found in the serum of patients with AIDS, and AIDS-related complex (Eyser *et al.*, 1983), and in culture supernatants of PBL cultured with influenza virus (Balkwill *et al.*, 1983) or corynebacterium parvum. LGL may produce it, as can B cells transformed by EBV (Revel and Schattner, 1987). It is not clear whether the gene producing acid-labile IFN-α is any of the known IFN-α genes, as the acid lability could be due to post-translational processing.

In sheep infected with maedi-visna virus, a retrovirus of the lentivirus family, the virus resides in monocytic cells. Recent studies have revealed that an atypical IFN is produced in sheep infected with this virus. This atypical IFN induced class II expression in normal sheep spleen and lymph node cells, which persisted for at least 2 weeks in the presence of the IFN. This IFN was non-glycosylated, of MW 54–64,000, and stable to heat and acid (Naroyan *et al.*, 1985; Kennedy *et al.*, 1985).

XV CONCLUSIONS

We have reviewed the involvement of IFN in autoimmune diseases, and because of personal interests have almost certainly overemphasized the role of IFN-γ compared to that of the other IFNs. Of particular interest is the acid-labile IFN-α, termed in a recent review of Michel Revel's "autoimmune interferon" (Revel and Schattner, 1987). This moiety is of considerable interest, but its role probably cannot be evaluated until it is cloned, its regulation is studied using cDNA probes, and its effects are compared with those of other IFNs by using pure material derived from expression of the cloned gene.

We have also focused on the role of IFN as an activator of pathological processes in autoimmunity. Because there is little information available we have not considered the possibility that a lack of the inhibitory, cytostatic influences of IFN-β, and especially IFN-β_2, may be of considerable importance.

A particular problem at the moment in the understanding of the role of molecular mediator in physiological or pathological processes is to untangle the "ripple" or "cascade" effects. The presence of a mediator, e.g. TNF, can induce another, e.g. IL-1, which in turn induces a third, e.g. PGE_2, IFN-β_2, and so on . . . Where does the cycle begin? It is important to understand more about the molecular interactions, so that we can devise efficient ways of controlling them. Another current problem is to understand the synergies (and antagonisms) of certain mediators. The synergy of IFN-γ with TNF is well documented, but it is unlikely to be the only example of this type, and synergies are likely to be of major importance in the pathogenesis of disease.

ACKNOWLEDGEMENTS

We thank our colleagues, both junior and senior, who are too numerous to list, for their contribution to our work and the development of these ideas over the past few years, the Arthritis and Rheumatism Council, ICI plc and Wellcome Trust for financial support, and Mrs P. Wells for preparing the manuscript.

REFERENCES

Abbott, R. J., Boderson, I. and Gruer, P. J. K. (1985). *Lancet* **ii**, 456–457.

Balkwill, F. R., Griffin, D. B., Band, H. A. and Beverley, P. C. L. (1983). *J. Exp. Med.* **157**, 1059–1063.

Bottazzo, G. F., Pujol-Borrell, R., Hanafusa, T. and Feldmann, M. (1983). *Lancet* **ii**, 1115–1119.

Bottazzo, G. F., Dean, B. M., McNally, J. M., McKay, E. A., Swift, P. G. F. and Gamble, D. R. (1985). *N. Eng. J. Med.* **313**, 353–360.

Buchan, G., Barrett, K., Maini, R. N. and Feldmann, M. (1987) (submitted).

Burman, P., Karlsson, F., Oberg, K. and Alm, G. (1985). *Lancet* **ii**, 100–101.

Collins, T., Korman, A. J., Wake, C. T. *et al.*, (1984). *PNAS* **81,** 4917–4921.

Eyser, E., Goedert, J., Man-Chin Poon and Prebble, O. (1983). *N. Eng. J. Med.* **304,** 583–586.

Feldmann, M., Doniach, D. and Bottazzo, G. F. (1985). *In* "Immunology of Rheumatic Diseases" (S. Gupta and N. Talal, eds), pp. 271–300. Plenum Press Inc.

Feldmann, M., Londei, M., de Berardinis, P., Essery, G. *et al.* (1986). *In* "Agents and Actions", Vol. 19 (in press).

Feldmann, M., Buchan, G., Kissonerghis, M., Portillo, G. *et al.* (1987). "Proceedings of CIBA Symposium on Autoimmunity" (in press).

Fentiman, I. S., Thomas, B. S., Balkwill, F. R., Rubens, R. D. and Hayward, J. L. (1985). *Lancet* **i**, 1166.

Foulis, A. and Farquarson, M. A. (1986). *Diabetes* **35,** 1215–1224.

Gresser, I. (1982). *In* "Interferon 4" (I. Gresser, ed.), pp. 95–127. Academic Press, London and N.Y.

Isenberg, D. A., Rowe, D., Shore, M., Novick, D. and Beverley, P. C. L. (1986). *Clin. Exp. Immunol.* **63**, 450–458.

Kelley, V. and Roths, J. B. (1982). *J. Immunol.* **129**, 923–925.

Kennedy, P., Narayan, N., Ghotbi, Z., Hopkins, J., Gendleman, H. and Clements, J. E. (1985). *J. Exp. Med.* **162**, 1970–1982.

Klareskog, L., Forsum, U. and Peterson, P. A. (1980). *Eur. J. Immunol.* **101**, 958–963.

Londei, M., Lamb, J. R., Bottazzo, G. F. and Feldmann, M. (1984). *Nature* **312**, 639–641.

Londei, M., Bottazzo, G. F. and Feldmann, M. (1985). *Science* **228**, 85–89.

Londei, M., Grubeck-Loebenstein, B., Greenall, C. and Feldmann, M. (1987a). *Acta Endocronologica* (in press).

Londei, M., Grubeck-Loebenstein, B., Kissonerghis, M. *et al.* (1987b). *Acta Endocronologica* (in press).

Martinez-Maza, O., Andersson, U., Andersson, J., Britton, S. and de Ley, M. (1984). *J. Immunol.* **132**, 251–255.

Massa, P. T., Dorries, R. and ter Meulen, V. (1986). *Nature* **320**, 543–546.

Naroyan, D., Sheffer, D., Clements, J. and Tennekoon, G. (1985). *J. Exp. Med.* **162**, 1954–1969.

Preble, O., Black, R., Friedman, R., Klippel, J. and Vilcek, J. (1982). *Science* **216**, 429–431.

Pujol-Borrell, R., Todd, I., Doshi, M., Bottazzo, G. F., Sutton, R., Gray, D., Adolf, G. R., Feldmann, M. (1987). *Nature* **326**, 304–306.

Pujol-Borrell, R., Todd, I., Doshi, M., Gray, D., Feldmann, M. and Bottazzo, G. F. (1986). *Clin. Exp. Immunol.* **65**, 128–139.

Revel, M. and Schattner, A. (1987). "CIBA Foundation Symposium on Autoimmunity" (in press).

Rhodes, J., Jones, D. and Bleheen, N. (1983). *Clin. Exp. Immunol.* **53**, 739–743.

Rhodes, J., Ivanyi, J. and Cozens, P. (1986). *Eur. J. Immunol.* **16**, 370–375.

Sobel, R. A. and Colwin, R. B. (1986). *J. Immunol.* **137**, 2132–2138.

Spies, T., Martin, C., Nedospasor, S., Fiers, W., Pious, D. and Strominger, J. (1986). *Proc. Natl Acad. Sci.* **83**, 8699–8702.

Taguchi, O., Takahashi, T., Seto, M., Namikawa, R., Matsuyama, M. and Nishizuka, Y. (1986). *J. Exp. Med.* **164**, 60–71.

Todd, I., Pujol-Borrell, R., Hammond, L. J., Bottazzo, G. F. and Feldmann, M. (1985). *Clin. Exp. Immunol.* **61**, 265–273.

Todd, I., Pujol-Borrell, R., Abdul-Karim, B. A. S., Hammond, L. J., Feldmann, M. and Bottazzo, G. F. (1987a). *Clin. Exp. Immunol.* (in press).

Todd, I., Pujol-Borrell, R., Hammond, L. J., McNally, J. M., Feldmann, M. and Bottazzo, G. F. (1987b). *Clin. Exp. Immunol.* (in press).

Ulrichs, K. and Muller-Rucholitz, W. (1985). *Diagnostic Immunology,* **3,** 47–55.

Ulrichs, K., Keller, R., Nothling, R., Schubert, G. and Muller-Rucholitz (1986). Presented at BSI, November 1986.

Walker, R., Cooke, A., Bone, A. J., Dean, B., Van der Meade, P., and Baird, J. D. (1986). *Diabetologia,* **29,** 749–751.

Wright, J. R., Lacy, P. E., Unanue, E. R., Mszynski, C. and Hamptfeld, V. (1986). *Diabetes* **35**, 1174–1177.

The Interferon–Interleukin 1 Connection

A. BILLIAU

Rega Institute for Medical Research, Katholieke Universiteit Leuven, B-3000 Leuven, Belgium.

The last two or three years have seen the demonstration of multiple interactions between interferons (IFNs) and other cytokines or their receptors. Examples are legion: synergistic actions between IFNs and other cytokines, effects on expression of receptors, induction of one cytokine by another, etc. In many instances these interactions allow for positive or negative feedback loops, the role of which in physiological and pathological processes is a matter of intensive current research.

INTERFERON 9
ISBN 0 12 302558 3

The concept that IFNs may be induced by endogenous mediators was first substantiated by the finding that the presence of interleukin 2 (IL-2) is a prerequisite for production of IFN-γ by T cells (Farrar *et al.*, 1981; Vilček *et al.*, 1985). At about the same time that this concept was introduced, observations done in my laboratory led us to postulate the existence of a leukocyte-derived cytokine which is able to induce normal fibroblasts to produce an IFN-β (Van Damme *et al.*, 1983a, b). It is now generally assumed that both IL-1 (Billiau *et al.*, 1985, 1986; Van Damme *et al.*, 1985a, b, 1987c) and TNF (Kohase *et al.*, 1986) possess this ability. Through the work of our laboratory and that of our colleagues in other Belgian Universities (Content *et al.*, 1985; Van Damme *et al.*, 1987a) it has also become known that these cytokines induce another protein which was formerly known as 26K protein or IFN-β_2 but which is in reality a potent growth factor for certain B-cell lines.

In this chapter I will describe how between 1980 and 1985 my collaborators and I, who had until then been studying the production, action and clinical applicability of IFN-β, came to work on IL-1 and came to demonstrate its potential to induce IFN-β and the B cell growth factor.

I INTERLEUKIN-1: AN INTRODUCTION

IL-1 (for reviews see Dinarello, 1984: Kampschmidt, 1984; Oppenheim *et al.*, 1986) is the name given in 1979 (Aarden *et al.*, 1979) to a monocyte-derived factor which had previously been described under different names such as lymphocyte activating factor (LAF), mitogenic protein (MP), helper peak-1 (HP-1), T cell replacing factor (TRF), B cell activating factor (BAF) and B cell differentiation factor (BDF). All these factors had been studied as possible mediators of antigen-specific immune reactions. Since all of them possessed similar physicochemical characteristics, a new name was introduced: interleukin-1.

Shortly thereafter it became clear that another series of factors which had been investigated in the framework of nonspecific host responses also had similar characteristics. These factors were: endogenous pyrogen (EP), leukocyte endogenous mediator (LEM), catabolin, and monocytic cell factor (MCF). EP (also called leukocytic pyrogen) was originally described as a factor released by granulocytes in response to endotoxin and various other stimuli, and was held responsible for the fever induced by microbial agents. LEM was originally defined as a similar leukocyte-derived factor that was held responsible for the so-called acute phase response, i.e. changes in the levels of proteins and minerals in the serum seen in acute infections and certain other acute pathological conditions. MCF is a factor defined by its ability to induce the release of collagenase, protease, and prostaglandins by synovial cells *in vitro* and is held responsible for tissue breakdown in arthritis. Catabolin was defined by its ability to cause systemic degradation of the musculoskeletal system.

These factors we originally described as being produced by leukocytes in response mainly to bacterial endotoxin but also to various other agents. The oldest of these factors is EP. It was originally believed to be a typical product of granulocytes. However, at about the time when the term IL-1 was introduced by immunologists, reports appeared indicating that EP and LEM are in fact products of monocytes that are indistinguishable from IL-1 (Murphy *et al.*, 1980; Sztein *et al.*, 1981). Hence, the inventory of biological activities assigned to IL-1 was enlarged to include EP, LEM, MCF and catabolin. More significant was the fact that IL-1 and its producer, the mononuclear phagocyte, had become the checkpoint where students of nonspecific and specific host responses had met.

Since then, several additional biological activities have been added to the IL-1 repertoire. In fact, the induction of IFN-β_1, discovered in our laboratory, is only one of them. The subsequent discovery that IL-1 also induces production of another protein (26K) to which antiviral activity had been assigned challenged our postulate that the antiviral effect of IL-1 was due to induction of IFN-β_1. Further work revealed that this protein is not an IFN but a growth factor for B cell hybridomas and plasmacytomas.

II "FIBROBLAST INTERFERON" HuIFN-β, HuIFN-β_1 and HuIFN-β_2

Our discovery of the IFN-β-inducing effect of IL-1 would not have occurred if it had not been for our previous experience and expertise with the production and purification of IFN-β from human fibroblasts (Billiau *et al.*, 1977, 1979; Heine *et al.*, 1981). HuIFN-β was formerly designated as fibroblast interferon, while HuIFN-α was called leukocyte interferon. These terms were introduced around 1970 simply to indicate the different cellular origins of the preparations: at that time there was no evidence that the active molecules in the preparations were physically or chemically different. Such evidence became available when it was demonstrated that antisera directed against fibroblast IFN did not neutralize leukocyte IFN and vice versa (Havell *et al.*, 1975). The current division of IFN into types α, β and γ is still essentially based on this lack of crossreactivity in seroneutralization reactions.

The classical procedure by which human fibroblasts are induced to produce HuIFN-β is by "superinduction". This consists in sequential exposure of the cells, over a period of 4–6 hours, to poly(I:C), cycloheximide and actinomycin D, following which the cells are washed, refed and reincubated for 16–24 hours. During this incubation a relatively large amont of IFN-β is produced.

Even with the new nomenclature, it is still correct to call a crude preparation of IFN-β from human fibroblasts "fibroblast interferon". The term IFN-β should indeed be reserved for designating the individual molecule or a pure preparation containing no other IFNs (e.g. α or γ) or other undefined impurities. One of the interesting impurities in crude human fibroblast IFN is a molecule called "26K" or IFN-β_2. This molecule was discovered independently in rather similar circumstances by Revel and colleagues at the Weizmann Institute, Rehovot, Israel (Weissenbach *et al*., 1979, 1980), and W. Fiers and colleagues and J. Content and colleagues, respectively at the State University of Gent and the Pasteur Institute in Brussels, Belgium (Content *et al*., 1982; Poupart *et al*., 1984). These investigators were using basically similar strategies to clone the gene of HuIFN-β. In the process of doing so techniques were needed to detect the translation product of the HuIFN-β mRNA. One of the techniques used consisted of translating poly(A)$^+$-rich RNAs extracted from superinduced fibroblasts in reticulocyte lysate and immunoprecipitating the translation products with antiserum (believed to be) specific for HuIFN-β. At the time when this was first being done, the best available antisera were found to precipitate two major translation products: a 17 and a 26 kD protein. Later on, more specific anti-HuIFN-β antisera became available that only precipitated the 17 kD protein. It would soon appear that this component was indeed the HuIFN-β protein. However, the 26 kD protein and its corresponding mRNA continued to arouse interest, mainly because the Weizmann Institute group found that this mRNA was translated by *Xenopus oocytes* into a secreted product possessing antiviral activity that was neutralizable by antisera directed against pure HuIFN-β.

cDNA clones of the 26 K mRNA were obtained and analysed (Weissenbach *et al*., 1980), and it was found that the amino acid sequence, as derived from the nucleic acid sequence, had no homology with that of any of the known human IFNs. Although serological cross-reactivity without sequence homology is not easily explained, the Weizmann investigators felt that the 26 kD protein fulfilled all the criteria for being called an IFN. Furthermore, since the types of IFN (α, β, γ) are defined on the basis of cross-neutralization reactions, they also felt that the 26 kD protein deserved the name HuIFN-β. Finally, to distinguish it from the classical HuIFN-β, they introduced the designations "HuIFN-β_1" for the classical HuIFN-β and "HuIFN-β_2" for the 26 kD protein.

A point of controversy between the Israeli and Belgian workers was that the latter refused to accept the designation of the molecule as IFN-β_2. Basically, their point was that: (1) they could not confirm that the 26 kD protein has antiviral activity at all; and (2) the sequence homology between the protein and classical HuIFN-β is too little to justify its classification as an IFN-β. While this work was going on in Israel and Belgium, evidence was also presented by workers from New York (Sehgal and Sagar, 1980) suggesting that there exist more than one mRNA species for HuIFN-β and that there might even exist several different genes.

Up to this point our own laboratory had played little part, except that we had provided the antisera to the Ghent group for the cloning of HuIFN-β. It is important, however, to note that the early antisera that we supplied were prepared against semi-purified fibroblast interferon (adsorption/desorption to controlled pore glass) and precipitated both the 17 kD (HuIFN-β) and the 26 kD proteins. Later antisera had been raised against IFN purified on Zn-chelate columns and these precipitated only the 17 kD (HuIFN-β) protein. Possessing these antisera and knowing the difference in specificity would prove to be of crucial importance for our future work.

III THE DISCOVERY OF ANOTHER IFN-β-LIKE ANTIVIRAL FACTOR IN "IMMUNE INTERFERON"

Around 1980, we developed an interest in IFN-γ, formerly called "immune interferon". This IFN is produced by treating suspensions of leukocytes with appropriate mitogens. In our laboratory we mostly used buffy coat-derived mononuclear cells induced with concanavalin A. Our primary objective was to obtain sufficient IFN-γ in pure form to study its physical, chemical and biological properties. Two difficulties had to be overcome: low yields in the production and a host of contaminants present in the crude starting product. Batches of crude immune IFN were submitted to a first rough concentration and purification step consisting of adsorption to silicic acid and desorption by ethylene glycol. Pools of this partially purified IFN were then further processed through several additional steps, the first of which was gel filtration.

Although this step worked reproducibly (De Ley *et al.*, 1980) and yielded a peak of IFN at $M_r = 45{,}000$, the recoveries were deplorably low: 90% or more of the biological activity seemed to be lost. Initially, we did not feel uneasy about this: loss of biological activity on purification is a phenomenon that interferonologists have learned to live with. However, as the recoveries did not improve with time, frustrations inevitably developed.

It so happened that two of my collaborators who worked on this project used different cells for their IFN assays: diploid cells in the production lab,

Hep-2 cells in the biochemistry laboratory. The possibility was therefore considered that low recoveries might be due to lesser sensitivity of the Hep-2 assay. However, this possibility was dismissed because the two laboratories used the same internal laboratory standard preparation. In this initial phase of our work, the standard preparation consisted of unpurified crude immune IFN. Accordingly, the titres of crude IFN batches, when standardized on this preparation, were independent of the assay systems. On the face of things it appeared as if 90% or more of the IFN was simply lost during fractionation by gel filtration. The enigma was solved when, after several months, the fractions of a gel filtration run were titrated not only on Hep-2 cells but also on diploid cells. It then became clear that antiviral activity on diploid cells was due to two components: one associated with a protein migrating at 45 kD (HuIFN-γ) and another migrating at 22 kD. By titration on Hep-2 cells only the 45 kD was detectable (Van Damme *et al.*, 1981).

IV THE INDUCER HYPOTHESIS

The observation that immune IFN contained a 22 kD antiviral factor (henceforth designated as 22K) demonstrable by assay on diploid cells, but not on Hep-2 cells, proved reproducible over more than 50 gel filtration runs. The question now arose as to what the nature of this material was. We quickly learned that its biological activity was acid-resistant and neutralizable by antisera directed against HuIFN-β. Accordingly we initially believed that it was some classical IFN-β coproduced with the IFN-γ by macrophages, monocytes or B cells. Nevertheless, we felt uneasy about the fact that this IFN did not act on Hep-2 cells which, according to previous experience, were not at all insensitive to classical HuIFN-β. One of the possibilities we considered was that our 22 K factor was identical with the molecule that the Weizmann Institute group had termed HuIFN-β_2. However, this material was at the time not available for comparative studies.

Therefore we had little alternative but to systematically study the physicochemical, biological and serological properties of the 22K factor. Since the factor seemed related to HuIFN-β, the first approach we considered worthwhile was to purify the factor with the two-step method that we had used for classical HuIFN-β: adsorption to silicic acid or CPG and elution by glycine at pH 2, followed by chromatography on Zn-chelate. In testing the feasibility of this scheme, we learned that, much like HuIFN-β, the 22K factor did adsorb to silicic acid and could indeed be eluted by acid. Hence, in this respect it did not differ from classical HuIFN-β. However, when the material was subsequently loaded on a Zn-chelate column its behaviour was found to be different in that it did not absorb. At first we did not take this observation very seriously, because we knew from previous experience that adsorption of proteins to metal chelate columns is a capricious process in itself. Nevertheless, this was a second hint that 22K and HuIFN-β were different molecules. The next indication came when we tried to use antibodies directed against HuIFN-β as an immunosorbent for the purification of the 22K antiviral factor. A column was used that had repeatedly proven to be effective in purification of classical HuIFN-β. Surprisingly, when 22K factor was loaded on this column it failed to adsorb. Yet the antiviral activity of the material which had failed to bind on the column was neutralizable by the same antibody that had been used to activate the column. This observation presented us with a paradox: how could the biological activity of protein be neutralized by an antibody without being bound by it? However, we were so preoccupied with finding a method to purify 22K that at first we attributed the unexpected result to some artefact in the functioning of the columns.

The next piece of evidence emerged when we succeeded in preparing an antibody against the 22K factor. Our primary purpose in obtaining this antibody was, again, to enable us to purify the factor by immuno-affinity. The main difficulty in obtaining the antibody consisted in making it so specific that it would not also bind or neutralize the main contaminant of 22K, namely IFN-γ. When we finally succeeded, the big surprise was that this antibody, while neutralizing the antiviral activity of 22K, did not neutralize the activity of classical HuIFN-β. So here was another paradox: anti-HuIFN-β neutralized 22K but anti-22K did not neutralize HuIFN-β.

At that time (mid-1982) we felt that we had enough material to write a decent paper which would describe our 22K factor as a "new β-like interferon". When my colleague Van Damme and I sat down to write this paper, it occurred to us that we would have to give evidence for 22K factor to meet the classical criteria required for any substance to qualify as an IFN: protein nature, broad antiviral spectrum, requirement for RNA and protein synthesis, etc. It was when writing these paragraphs that Van Damme considered the possibility that 22K factor might be an inducer of IFN rather than an IFN. In fact, we had briefly contemplated this possibility early during our work, even before we had all the paradoxical results described above. However, for some reason we had forgotten this inducer hypothesis. Now, facing the problem of having to write down our arguments, the possibility resurfaced. I especially remember one episode that occurred one Friday evening after we had sat down together again, encouraging each other to finish up the manuscript. Van Damme said suddenly: "Whatever I write, I cannot exclude the possibility that 22K is an inducer rather than an interferon!" As I wanted to finish the discussion and go home for the weekend I reacted: "Well, why don't you write that it *is* an inducer!" The idea remained with us during the weekend and on Monday morning we had a new series of discussions which led to the rewriting of our manuscript. It now occurred to us that all paradoxes were easily resolved. When the text was ready we showed it to De Somer, then the ultimate test in our Institute for an idea to make sense. In his usual way he snapped: "It's a nice idea and a nice paper, but you won't be able to sell it. Besides, there is an easy way to prove your hypothesis: show that cells make interferon if you treat them with 22K." As a result of De Somer's comments we rewrote the paper, diplomatically leaving open the two possibilities: (1) 22K is a new β-related IFN and (2) 22K is an inducer of IFN-β. After some misadventures the paper did get accepted for publication (Van Damme *et al.*, 1983b).

At about the time when the manuscript was completed, the International Congress of Interferon took place in Miami, Florida (November, 1982). I presented our data and formulated the two hypotheses, with a clear preference for the inducer alternative. I also spent some time explaining to the audience the difficulty of distinguishing between an IFN and an inducer of IFN using an antiviral assay. I compared the antiviral effect measured in the bioassay with the shadows on the wall of Plato's cave, leaving those who watch the shadows with the task of defining the shape of the real objects that cast them. Our colleague, Jan Vilček, was in the audience and reacted sympathetically by appreciating the poetry of that image, but expressed the opinion that a few well-designed experiments should allow us to make the distinction.

On my way back from the Miami meeting I happened to travel in the same plane with some Belgian friends, including Jean Content. He suggested that looking at the mRNA for IFN-β in cells treated with 22K might allow us to provide positive proof of the inducer hypothesis. In fact, we had already attempted to do some experiments along this line, in which we had extracted mRNA from 22K-induced cells and tried to translate this RNA into bioactive HuIFN-β in oocytes. Content insisted that, using his probes, he might have a better chance. This episode led to a series of collaborative experiments that would eventually prove our point. However, before discussing these experiments I must first describe the identification of the 22K factor as being nothing else than IL-1.

V 22K: A PHANTASM?

Although we had no definitive proof, we felt at ease with our inducer hypothesis. All our data could now be nicely fitted together. Meanwhile we had also learned that 22K did not bind to immobilized ConA, suggesting that, in contrast to HuIFN-β, it was not glycosylated. We had also found that its biological activity was resistant to treatment with SDS.

It was clear that now we had to put all our efforts into the isolation of pure 22K, so that its molecular nature could be elucidated. At about that time (mid-1983) our regular purification scheme called for: (1) batch adsorption to silicic acid and elution by EG; (2) batch adsorption of impurities to DEAE-Sephacel; and (3) gel filtration and collection of the 22K fractions. We then started applying a fourth step: cation exchange on FPLC. My collaborator, Marc De Ley, had successfully been using this method to purify 45K Hu-IFN-γ, and he was eager to adapt the conditions for purification of 22K. After several runs he obtained active fractions in which he could not detect any protein by the methods then used in our laboratory. For instance, when using SDS-PAGE, no stainable protein bands would appear. Our interpretation was that all impurities had been removed, but that there was too little of the 22K protein itself for it to show up on the SDS gels. But De Somer's interpretation was quite different: "Are you sure you are not dealing with a spook?" This question of his was not without grounds. Over and over again, ever since our work on 22K had started, we had passed through episodes of weeks or months during which the antiviral activity of 22K became undetectable. Moreover, in episodes when the titrations *did* work, we mostly failed to obtain nice dose–response curves. Typically, viral CPE would be inhibited by 50% at the endpoint dilution, but with higher concentrations protection would reach 60–70%, but not 100%. De Somer was aware of all this. The negative episodes in which we simply could not do any experiments irritated him, and he had decided that 22K was just complex biological activity, in other words a spook on which we should not risk our reputations.

My advice to my collaborators was: "Stick to your guns", which they did. Late in 1983 Van Damme collected the material of about 10 gel filtration runs, representing buffy coats from about 500 blood donations, and supplied them to De Ley to be purified by FPLC. The active fraction was analysed again by SDS-PAGE. Then the spook appeared as a unique 17.5 kD band on the gel. It took two more experiments to confirm that the biological activity coincided with the stained band. We felt that we had purified our 22K factor to electrophoretic homogeneity.

Since, apparently, the 22K preparations were electrophoretically homogeneous, it was logical to try and determine the *N*-terminal amino acid sequence. For this we enlisted the expert help of our colleague Van Beeumen at the State University of Ghent. On April 12, 1984 an exhilarated Van Damme stepped into my office and proudly showed me a sequence of seven amino acids. Four days later we had 39. Two additional runs on similar preparations were done. By and large they confirmed the first sequence, but also showed that the preparation was not quite homogeneous yet, in that minor signals repeatedly showed up at some positions. One thing was sure, however: 22K was not a spook, unless some spooks have amino acid sequences.

VI REDISCOVERING IL-1

The fact that 22K had a consistent amino acid sequence gave us confidence that it truly existed. But we still did not know what its real biological significance was. The fact that it could induce IFN-β did not yet mean that that was its real function in the organism. Moreover, as explained above, the IFN-inducing potential of 22K was marginal: (1) only certain cells responded; (2) dose–response curves were often not clear-cut; and (3) the antiviral effect sometimes became undetectable for several weeks in a row. Thus, the spook-like properties of 22K suggested to us that, *in vivo*, it might have a quite different function. The implication of this was that instead of having discovered a new factor, we might have rediscovered an old one. Although this possibility had been on our minds ever since we had been working on 22K, it had not been of much concern until we had the *N*-terminal amino acid sequence. Our sequence was not present in any of the amino-acid sequence banks and we had not come across it in the recent lymphokine and monokine literature. But we thought it very likely that somewhere, somebody was working on the same molecule and would one day produce the same sequence.

A Skin-Reactive Factor?

In the late 1970s we had seen that intracutaneous injection of fibroblast IFN caused a local inflammatory response that showed some resemblance to a delayed type hypersensitivity reaction (DTH) (De Somer *et al.*, 1977). Also, in the literature a lymphokine or monokine is described, called SRF (skin reactive factor) which is held to be responsible for the DTH-skin response (Bloom, 1971). The factor was poorly characterized, but it seemed possible that 22K as well as IFN-β might have something to do with the phenomenon. Therefore, in early 1981 De Somer and I both injected ourselves with 0.1 ml of a 22K preparation purified to the stage of gel filtration. After about 6 hours the injection site started itching and swelling. The following day redness developed. The reaction was much stronger than we had ever seen before with similar injections of classical HuIFN-β. After 48 hours the reaction subsided but some discoloration indicated that extravasation had taken place.

Subsequently, Van Damme did some experiments in rabbits, in which he injected all the fractions of a gel filtration run. Some fractions caused an immediate inflammation, but only those coinciding with the 22K antiviral peak gave a delayed type reaction. Nevertheless, we were not sure that the reactions were due to the 22K antiviral factor, because the preparations we then had available were still grossly heterogeneous. In later experiments with homogeneous 22K, skin reaction in rabbits, although still present, was much less pronounced. Biopsies of such rabbits revealed extensive granulocyte infiltration, and this would later lead us to think about chemotaxis and possible effects on redistribution of blood leukocytes.

B Lymphotoxin?

Although 22K preparations of various degrees of purity had neither outright toxic effects nor growth inhibitory effects on cells, we could not refute the possibility that apparent antiviral effects and/or induction of IFN-β could be properties of lymphotoxin, and hence that 22K might fall into that category of factors. Late in 1983, we sent semi-purified as well as electrophoretically homogeneous 22K to our colleague Jan Vilček, whom we knew was intensively working on lymphotoxins. His answer was clear: the crude and semi-pure preparations did have lymphotoxin activity; the homogeneous 22K was devoid of such activity. We decided that 22K was not a classical lymphotoxin.

C Colony-Stimulating Factor?

Early in 1984, as I tried to recollect literature data on possible endogenous inducers of IFN, I vaguely remembered a conversation with my friend Jos Van der Meer of Leiden University in which he told me of studies by Rabinowitz (Fleit and Rabinovitch, 1981) showing that CSF is an inducer of IFN. I remember reacting rather sceptically. I called van der Meer and he gave me the exact literature reference. As it turned out, the observation was of some sort of priming rather than of an inducer effect of CSF preparations. Nevertheless, we decided to investigate the matter. Van Damme and I went to see Van der Meer, having in our coolbox a set of samples of 22K. Van der Meer explained to us all about CSFs, but we decided that he could not help us any further since he was working on mice, and 22K, according to the antiviral assay, was only active on human cells. Fortunately, in a neighbouring building Wim Fibbe of the Leiden hacmatology group was regularly doing human CSF assays. After less than two weeks we got the answer: positive. We would have liked to believe that 22K was no more or no less than one of the CSFs. But Fibbe was more critical, explaining that he could not exclude the possibility that 22K was in fact an inducer of CSF rather than being CSF itself. As it turned out, the hypothesis of our Leiden colleagues was correct: 22K induces monocytes in the bone marrow cultures to produce CSF and thereby indirectly stimulates bone marrow colonies to grow (Fibbe *et al.*, 1986).

D IL-1?

1 Monocytic cell factor

The first time I thought of IL-1 as being the identity behind the 22K mask was at the Roussel-UCLAF Round Table meeting on lymphokines in Paris on 23–24 February 1984. It was here that I first reported having isolated electrophoretically homogeneous 22K and that, also for the first time, I refuted all other alternatives to the IFN-inducer hypothesis. At the meeting, virtually all canonized monokines and lymphokines were reviewed by several presenters. At each presentation of another cytokine I tried to find arguments to identify it as our 22K factor. Most of all, I was struck by the presentation of J. F. Dayer of Geneva on monocytic cell factor (MCF), a monokine defined by its ability to induce collagenase and prostaglandin synthesis in synovial cells (Dayer *et al.*, 1979). Dayer explained that this factor was related if not identicial to IL-1. His thesis was that IL-1 was in reality not an interleukin in the true sense, because it has as many effects outside the immune system as within: aside from the effect on synovial cells, he mentioned effects on hepatocytes (amyloid release) and fever. So here was a monokine with various effects. Why would it not also have IFN-inducing potential? Furthermore, all the physicochemical properties fitted those of 22K. After the session I talked briefly with Dayer and he agreed to do some tests on our preparations.

After my return from the meeting, I hastened to send some 22K samples to the Geneva group. The answer came promptly. They had never seen an MCF preparation more active than our 22K.

2 Endogenous pyrogen

In April 1984 Ghislain Opdenakker of our laboratory had the idea of injecting 22K intravenously into a rabbit, mainly to check its effects on white blood cell counts. Opdenakker, a medical doctor, had been assisting Van Damme with the skin reactions and biopsies. Probably it was the granulocyte infiltrates in skin biopsies as well as the CSF results from the Leiden laboratory which gave him the idea of checking the haematological effects of 22K. The results were striking: 22K injection caused an immediate fall in granulocyte as well as lymphocyte counts (Van Damme *et al.*, 1986). After 6 hours the counts would increase again to normal and even supranormal values. These results were extensively discussed with De Somer who took his Topley and Wilson manual to show us that the effect was characteristic of endotoxin. From there to endogenous pyrogen (EP) was but a small step.

Classically, EP has been reported to cause an increase rather than a decrease in blood cell counts. As it turned out, this discrepancy with our data was merely a matter of dose. We had been injecting a dose that was probably higher than anybody had ever been able to do before. Therefore we saw a drastic decrease in leukocytes followed by an increase. In later experiments we would inject less 22K and find the classical increase, not preceded by a decrease (Van Damme *et al.*, 1986).

The next thing to do was to perform a few well controlled experiments to test the inherent pyrogenicity of 22K. Sure enough these experiments were consistent with 22K being related to or identical with EP.

3 LAF

It was now quite clear that, without really trying, we had landed right in the IL-1 field. It thus became imperative to test whether 22K had LAF-activity. The nearest laboratory where LAF tests were being done was that of Scandené in the Université Libre de Bruxelles, who agreed to run some tests on our 22K. The test was positive but, due to some linguistic problem, the quantitative aspect was misinterpreted by us. Apparently the sample had been tested undiluted. The positive result meant that there was more than 1 unit of LAF. In communicating with the Brussels scientists we had understood that there was *not* more than 1 unit of LAF. This result kept us in disarray for the whole summer, when finally we decided to have additional LAF tests done. This revealed that our 22K preparations had in fact unprecedented high LAF activity.

Even before we had resolved this difficulty, we felt that we had enough data to relate our amino acid sequence to the 22K antiviral effect and to EP, not to mention to possible MCF and CSF activities. Hence, in midsummer 1984 we submitted a manuscript to *Nature* (Van Damme *et al.*, 1985a). Meanwhile we anxiously watched the literature for IL-1-related sequences. We had been told that a person deeply involved in IL-1 cloning was Charles Dinarello of Tufts University in Boston. On the same day that we submitted out manuscript to *Nature*, I wrote to him, explaining our 22K problem and offering to exchange sequence data. Although our colleague was personally inclined to exchange sequence data, a *de visu* confrontation of sequences proved to be a process fraught with difficulties. It would take until late November (1st International Workshop on Interleukin-1 at Stifford near Grays, UK) for us to be allowed a quick glance at the sequence of the cDNA clone (Van Damme *et al.*, 1985c). This clone possessed a coding region predicting a protein of 31 kD, much too large for IL-1. However, our *N*-terminal sequence was 60% homologous with a stretch in the middle of this protein, consistent with the proposal (Auron *et al.*, 1984) that biologically active 17 kD IL-1 protein is derived from a 31 kD precursor.

VII IS THE 22K ANTIVIRAL FACTOR IDENTICAL TO IL-1?

The *N*-terminal sequence which we determined on a preparation of the 22K factor (Van Damme *et al.*, 1985a) was homologous with but not quite identical to that derived from the nucleic acid sequence of the IL-1 cDNA clone that became known shortly afterwards (Auron *et al.*, 1984). Since at that time there was already general agreement that there existed more than one molecule endowed with IL-1 activities, one of the possibilities that we had to consider was that our sequence represented one of the "other" IL-1s. On the other hand, we also remembered that when we did the amino acid sequencing some of the positions had been uncertain and that we had had to choose between several possible amino acids. Therefore, as soon as the cDNA sequence became available, we went back to the original chromatograms of the amino-acid analysis and, sure enough, we could detect all the signals corresponding to the cDNA-sequence. From this we concluded that IL-1 molecules corresponding to the cDNA sequence were certainly present in our preparations, but also that there was contamination by other proteins. Whether these proteins were irrelevant impurities or "other" IL-1 molecules was at that time not clear.

Since our primary purpose was not so much to analyse the possible heterogeneity of IL-1, but rather to establish the principle that there exist natural cytokines that act antivirally by inducing IFN-β, we did not make further attempts to purify or sequence our factor, but we decided to make our point by demonstrating that antiviral activity was a property of IL-1 preparations obtained by other investigators, and in particular of cloned IL-1. As expected, we found that these preparations possessed antiviral activity (Billiau *et al.*, 1986). Moreover, in all instances, this activity was neutralizable by antisera against HuIFN-β, supporting our contention that these molecules acted by inducing IFN-β.

Meanwhile, the sequence of another IL-1 (now called IL-1α) became known (March *et al.*, 1985) and it turned out to be quite different from the first one (now called IL-1β). This, as well as the fact that there exists only a single gene for IL-1β, told us that the aberrant amino acids in our original sequence of 22K factor had been due to irrelevant contaminants. We thus concluded that the antiviral factor which we had been calling 22K factor was in reality IL-1β.

VIII DOES IL-1 ACT ANTIVIRALLY BY INDUCING HuIFN-β_1, OR HuIFN-β_2 (26K PROTEIN)?

Having established beyond any doubt that the IFN-β-like 22K antiviral factor was in fact an IL-1, we still lacked formal proof that it acted by inducing production of IFN-β. In fact, we started doing experiments to provide such proof even before we knew that 22K was IL-1. The main difficulty was that when we treated cells with 22K factor (which henceforth I will call IL-1) we mostly failed to demonstrate significant secretion of IFN-β by the cells. If we concentrated the supernatant fluid, small amounts were found. However, amounts that were only slightly less also occurred in supernatants from untreated cells. Using the well-known trick of adding cycloheximide and actinomycin D did not help, as it caused an increase in background IFN-β production as well.

We then decided to turn to a search for increases in the levels of IFN-β mRNA in cells treated with IL-1 (Van Damme *et al.*, 1985b). As a means to detect the mRNA, we first used translation in oocytes. Later on, with the collaboration of Jean Content, we switched to RNA–DNA hybridization techniques. With both techniques we found that treatment of cells with IL-1 caused appearance of IFN-β mRNA levels that in most experiments were slightly above background. If IL-1 was used in combination with cycloheximide the levels of IFN-β mRNA were distinctly higher than with cycloheximide alone. Although we were not completely satisfied with these results, we felt that they did support our contention that the antiviral effect of IL-1 was due to induction of IFN-β. However, these experiments also led us to the observation that IL-1, although a weak inducer of IFN-β, was a potent inducer of the 26 kD protein. The observation was first made by Jean Content (Content *et al.*, 1985) who happend to have a longstanding interest in this protein. He took advantage of the availability of the dot-blot filters prepared for hybridization with the IFN-β probe. After washing them, he re-used the filters in hybridization runs with a 26 kD cDNA probe that he had available. It now became clear to him that IL-1 was the most potent inducer of the 26 kD mRNA that he had ever had in his hands.

Although the cDNA had been cloned and sequenced both in the laboratories of Michel Revel (Weissenbach *et al.*, 1980) and of Walter Fiers, the sequence information had remained unpublished for several years (Haegeman *et al.*, 1986; Revel *et al.*, 1986). Also, the biological function of the protein continued to be a matter of controversy. As explained earlier, the Israeli workers had assigned IFN-like antiviral activity to the protein and had coined the term IFN-β_2 for it. Our discovery that IL-1 was a potent inducer of this protein now presented us with the possibility that the antiviral effect of IL-1 would be due to induction of the 26 kD (IFN-β_2) protein rather than the classical IFN-β. For several reasons we remained reluctant to accept this explanation. In particular, together with Walter Fiers we felt that there was insufficient confirmed evidence that the 26 kD protein: (1) had antiviral effect; and (2) that neutralization of this antiviral effect by highly specific sera against classical IFN-β was due to direct binding of the protein and not to some other artefactual phenomenon.

To prove our point we felt that we needed an antibody against pure 26 kD protein that would not react with classical IFN-β. If such an antibody would not neutralize the antiviral effect of IL-1, while antisera against classical IFN-β did neutralize the effect, proof of our hypothesis would be complete. To raise the anti-26 kD antibody we had to prepare a suitable antigen and to develop an adequate assay system. As a source for 26 kD protein we used batches of semi-purified human fibroblast IFN that had been left over from several years earlier when they were being prepared for use in clinical trials. We knew that this IFN contained 26 kD protein because it had served as the antigen to prepare the polyspecific sera with which Walter Fiers and his group had first discovered the existence of the 26 kD mRNA. Therefore, my colleague Marc De Ley set out to purify the 26 kD protein from the old batches of fibroblast IFN. He used several strategies, including removal of the classical IFN-β by adsorption to Zn-chelate, followed by immunoaffinity chromatography to the polyspecific anti-IFN-β-antibody and FPLC. In so doing he isolated a protein peak fraction that contained a 26 kD protein which was immunoprecipitable with the polyspecific serum. However, he had no way of proving that this material was identical to the 26 kD protein that Walter Fiers had cloned. The reason for this was that we did not possess a suitable assay system. Nevertheless, our colleague decided to use his peak fraction for immunizing a rabbit. Because of the uncertainty with respect to their specificity, these sera were initially not used for experiments. Much later it would turn out that my colleague had made a good guess: his serum was monospecific for 26 kD, and although it did neutralize the biological activity of 26 kD protein it did not prevent the antiviral action of IL-1 (Van Damme *et al.*, 1987c), thereby eliminating the possibility that the antiviral effect of IL-1 is due to induction of 26 kD protein. However, we did these experiments only after we had been able to assess the specificity of the sera. This assessment only became possible at a point when we discovered the true biological function of 26 kD, i.e. growth-promoting activity for B cells.

IX 26 kD PROTEIN (ALIAS IFN-β_2): A B CELL GROWTH FACTOR

In mid-1985, in the midst of our concern to find a biological function for 26 kD, we received a call from our colleague Jacques Van Snick of the Ludwig Institute, Brussels branch. A specialist in B cell function, Van Snick had found that certain mouse T cell lines spontaneously release a factor which promotes the growth of mouse/rat hybridomas (Van Snick *et al.*, 1986). He considered the remote possibility that this factor might be an interleukin or an interferon and he asked us whether we could help him to test this possibility by providing IL-1 and/or IFN-containing preparations to test this possibility. Among the preparations that we supplied there was some crude NDV-induced L929-cell IFN, as well as a corresponding mock preparation. It turned out that the L929-cell IFN was very potent in his assay for hybridoma growth factor (HGF). By using antisera we quickly learned that this HGF activity was not due to the the IFN-α and -β in the preparation, but rather to a protein that was co-induced with the IFN. This observation spurred us to test whether the human 26 kD protein, that is a similarly co-induced protein, would possess HGF activity. A series of tests showed that all 26 kD protein-containing preparations had elevated HGF activity. In particular, crude as well as semi-purified preparations of human fibroblast IFN, obtained by superinduction, contained high levels of HGF. In contrast, pure IFN-β was completely devoid of activity. Most significant of all was our finding that HGF could be induced in fibroblasts by simple treatment with IL-1 (Van Damme *et al.*, 1987a, b). Doses as small as 0.1 antiviral unit/ml were found sufficient to cause measurable HGF production. At optimal doses of IL-1, yields of 10^4 units of HGF could be obtained. Close examination of the conditions required for induction of HGF revealed that they parallelled those required for induction of the 26 kD protein mRNA. Hence it was only logical to hypothesize that the 26 kD protein was the substance behind HGF.

To prove that the 26 kD protein and HGF were the same, we followed two lines of investigation. On the one hand, we undertook to isolate mRNA for HGF and show that it hybridized to 26 kD cDNA probes. On the other hand, we undertook to obtain IL-1-induced HGF in pure form and determine its *N*-terminal amino acid sequence. Both lines of investigation gave us positive evidence and thereby established beyond any doubt that the 26 kD protein was HGF (Van Damme *et al.*, 1987a).

X RELATION BETWEEN ANTIVIRAL AND B CELL GROWTH-PROMOTING ACTIVITIES OF THE 26 kD PROTEIN

The question of the true biological activity of the 26 kD protein had been a subject of controversy ever since 1980, when the protein was first described. As explained earlier, Revel and his coworkers assigned IFN-like activity to the molecule and designated it as IFN-β_2 (Weissenbach *et al.*, 1979).

Since, in the course of 1985, we had become more and more involved in the role of 26K as a possible mediator of the antiviral effects of IL-1, we wanted to verify whether or not it had antiviral activity. For one thing, our preparations were all devoid of activity. However, in the course of 1985, Dr Ruggieri from the Weizmann Institute visited our laboratory and it was agreed that we would receive some samples of 26 kD (IFN-β_2) protein derived from CHO-cells into which the 26 kD cDNA had been introduced. The tests were positive and we were happy to be able to inform our Israeli colleagues that we did find the expected amount of antiviral activity. Several months later, when we had obtained evidence for identity between 26 kD and the IL-1-induced HGF, we retrieved samples and found that they also contained high concentrations of HGF activity. Significantly, the titre of HGF activity exceeded that of antiviral activity by a 1000-fold factor.

It seemed reasonable to conclude from our results that the antiviral effect of 26 kD protein is little more than a side-effect and that the denomination "IFN-β_2" which refers to this side-effect should be abandoned. Most cytokines carry names that reflect their principal biological and physiological action. Our observation that the 26 kD protein is a potent HGF suggests that its function in the body may consist in promoting growth of certain B cell populations. Experiments by our colleagues at the Brussels Ludwig Institute to identify our HGF with known B cell growth or differentiation factors have so far yielded negative results. Conversely, it could be shown that the protein promotes *in vitro* growth of several mouse plasmacytomas (Van Damme *et al.,* 1987a), which otherwise can only be propagated by *in vivo* passage, indicating that 26K, if not important in B cell physiology, does play a role in B cell pathology.

The known natural inducers of the 26K protein are IL-1 (Content *et al.*, 1985) and TNF (Van Damme *et al.,* 1987a). Both these cytokines have been shown to promote growth of normal fibroblasts, although they are cytotoxic for certain continuous cell lines. While investigating the involvement of IFNs in the growth-promoting effect of TNF, Jan Vilček and coworkers found that polyclonal antisera directed against IFN-β could not block the effect (Kohase *et al.*, 1986). In contrast, they found that the anti-IFN-β antisera possessed growth-promoting effect for normal diploid fibroblasts. Hence, the suggestion was made that IFN-β production, occurring as a result of TNF treatment, served as a negative feedback control in growth regulation by TNF. In view of these data, growth enhancement seen in hybridoma and plasmacytoma cells may represent a pathological rather than a physiological response to the 26 kD protein, whose real physiological function might consist in inhibiting rather than stimulating, growth of cells. Obviously, confirmation of this hypothesis would provide an entirely new insight into such phenomena as wound-healing, in which positive as well as negative cell growth regulation play a crucial role. Even more significantly, it would also substantiate the concept that some forms of malignant conversion of cells may result from the fact that their receptors for growth-inhibitory cytokines are aberrant in that they are connected to intracellular pathways that are growth-promoting rather than growth-inhibitory.

An important question is that of the universality of the 26 kD protein. Production of HGF is not the prerogative of fibroblasts or fibroblastoid cells. In fact, several authors before us described similar HGF activity produced by other cells, in particular monocytes (Aarden *et al.*, 1985) and endothelial cells (Astaldi *et al.*, 1980). Also, our colleagues from the Brussels Ludwig Institute isolated T cell lines of mice which produce HGF (Van Snick *et al.*, 1986). Do all these factors represent the activities of a single molecular type or is there a family of related molecules with HGF activity? As yet there is little information on this issue, except that we found a close serological relationship between the human fibroblast-derived HGF (26K) and the HGF that is produced by peripheral blood leucocytes in response to mitogen stimulation (Van Damme *et al.*, 1987b).

By assigning a role to the 26 kD protein as a growth regulator and by establishing a convenient and sensitive biological assay system, our work has provided the conceptual and technical keys that were needed to open the mysterious black box that "26K" once stood for.

ACKNOWLEDGEMENTS

This story is a tribute to my close collaborators, Jo Van Damme, Ghislain Opdenakker and Mark de Ley as well as to our fellow workers in Belgium, Jean Content of the Pasteur Institute of Brabant and Jacques Van Snick of the Ludwig Institute in Brussels. Last but not least I dedicate my narrative to my mentor Piet De Somer who unfortunately died in 1985.

REFERENCES

Aarden, L. A., Brunner, T. K., Cerottini, J.-C., Dayer, J.-M., de Weck, A. L., Dinarello, C. A., Di Sabato, G., Farrar, J. J., Gery, I., Gillis, S., Handschumacher, R. E., Henney, C. S., Hoffmann, M. K., Koopman, W. J., Krane, S. M., Lachman, L. B., Lefkowits, I., Mishell, R. I., Mizel, S. B., Oppenheim, J. J., Paetkau, V., Plate, J., Röllinghoff, M., Rosenstreich, D., Rosenthal, A. S., Rosenwasser, L. J., Schimpl, A., Shin, H. S., Simon, P. L., Smith, K. A., Wagner, H., Watson, J. D., Wecker, E. and Wood, D. D. (1979). *J. Immunol.* **123**, 2928–2929.

Aarden, L., Lansdorp, P. and De Groot, E. (1985). *In* "Lymphokines" (E. Pick and M. Landy, eds), vol. 10, pp. 175–185. Academic Press, London and New York.

Astaldi, G. C. B., Janssen, M. C., Lansdorp, P., Willems, C., Zeijlemaker, W. P. and Oosterhof, F. (1980). *J. Immunol.* **125**, 1411–1414.

Auron, P. E., Webb, A. C., Rosenwasser, L. J., Mucci, S. F., Rich, A., Wolff, S. M. and Dinarello, C. A. (1984). *Proc. Natl Acad. Sci. USA* **81**, 7907–7911.

Billiau, A., Edy, V. G., Heremans, H., Van Damme, J., Desmyter, J., Georgiades, J. and De Somer, P. (1977). *Antimicrob. Agents Chemother.* **12**, 11–15.

Billiau, A., Van Damme, J., Van Leuven, F., Edy, V. G., De Ley, M., Cassiman, J.-J., Van Den Berghe, H. and De Somer, P. (1979). *Antimicrob. Agents Chemother.* **16**, 49–55.

Billiau, A., Opdenakker, G., Van Damme, J., De Ley, M., Volckaert, G. and Van Beeumen, J. (1985). *Immunol. Today* **6**, 235–236.

Billiau, A., Van Damme, J., Opdenakker, G., Fibbe, W. E., Falkenburg, J. H. F. and Content, J. (1986). *Immunobiol.* **172**, 323–335.

Bloom, B. R. (1971). *Adv. Immunol.* **13**, 101–208.

Cameron, P., Limjuco, G., Rodkey, J., Bennett, C. and Schmidt, J. A. (1985). *J. Exp. Med.* **162**, 790–801.

Content, J., De Wit, L., Pierard, D., Derynck, R., De Clercq, E. and Fiers, W. (1982). *Proc. Natl Acad. Sci. USA* **79**, 2768–2772.

Content, J., De Wit, L., Poupart, P., Opdenakker, G., Van Damme, J. and Billiau, A. (1985). *Eur. J. Biochem.* **152**, 253–257.

Dayer, J. M., Bréard, J., Chess, L. and Krane, S. M. (1979). *J. Clin. Invest.* **64**, 1386–1392.

De Ley, M., Van Damme, J., Claeys, H., Weening, H., Heine, J. W., Billiau, A., Vermylen, C. and De Somer, P. (1980). *Eur. J. Immunol.* **10**, 877–883.

De Somer, P., Edy, V. G. and Billiau, A. (1977). *Lancet* **ii**, 47–48.

Dinarello, C. A. (1984). *Rev. Infect. Dis.* **6**, 51–95.

Farrar, W. L., Johnson, H. M. and Farrar, J. J. (1981) *J. Immunol.* **126,** 1120–1125.

Fibbe, W. E., Van Damme, J., Billiau, A., Voogt, P. J., Duinkerken, N., Kluck, P. M. C. and Falkenburg, J. H. F. (1986). *Blood* **68,** 1316–1321.

Fleit, H. B. and Rabinovitch, M. (1981). *Cell. Immunol.* **57**, 495–504.

Haegeman, G., Content, J., Volckaert, G., Derynck, R., Tavernier, J. and Fiers, W. (1986). *Eur. J. Biochem.* **159,** 625–632.

Havell, E. A., Berman, B., Ogburn, C. A., Berg, K., Paucker, K. and Vilček, J. (1975). *Proc. Natl Acad. Sci. USA* **72**, 2185–2187.

Heine, J. W., Van Damme, J., De Ley, M., Billiau, A. and De Somer, P. (1981). *J. Gen. Virol.* **54**, 47–56.

Kampschmidt, R. F. (1984). *J. Leukocyte Biol.* **36**, 341–355.

Kohase, M. Henriksen-De Stefano, D., May, L. T., Vilček, J. and Sehgal, P. B. (1986). *Cell* **45**, 659–669.

March, C. J., Mosley, B., Larsen, A., Cerretti, D. P., Braedt, G., Price, V., Gillis, S., Henney, C. S., Kronheim, S. R., Grabstein, K., Conlon, P. J., Hopp, T. P. and Cosman, D. (1985). *Nature* **315**, 641–647.

Murphy, P. A., Simon, P. L. and Willoughby, W. F. (1980). *J. Immunol.* **124**, 2498–2501.

Oppenheim, J. J., Kovacs, E. J., Matsushima, K. and Durum, S. K. (1986). *Immunol. Today* **7**, 45–56.

Poupart, P., De Wit, L. and Content, J. (1984). *Eur. J. Biochem.* **143**, 15–21.

Revel, M., Ruggieri, R. and Zilberstein, A. (1986). *In* "The Biology of the Interferon System 1985" (H. Schellekens and W. E. Stewart II, eds), pp. 207–216. Elsevier, Amsterdam.

Sehgal, P. B. and Sagar, A. D. (1980). *Nature* **288**, 95–98.

Sztein, M. B., Vogel, S. N., Sipe, J. D., Murphy, P. A., Mizel, S. B., Oppenheim, J. J. and Rosenstreich, D. L. (1981). *Cell. Immunol.* **63**, 164–176.

Van Damme, J., De Ley, M., Claeys, H., Billiau, A., Vermylen, C. and De Somer, P. (1981). *Eur. J. Immunol.* **11**, 937–942.

Van Damme, J., Billiau, A., De Ley, M. and De Somer, P. (1983a). *In* "The Biology of the Interferon System 1983" (E. De Maeyer and H. Schellekens, eds), pp. 153–158. Elsevier, Amsterdam.

Van Damme, J., Billiau, A., De Ley, M. and De Somer, P. (1983b). *J. Gen. Virol.* **64**, 1819–1822.

Van Damme, J., De Ley, M., Opdenakker, G., Billiau, A., De Somer, P. and Van Beeumen, J. (1985a). *Nature* **314**, 266–268.

Van Damme, J., Opdenakker, G., Billiau, A., De Somer, P. De Wit, L., Poupart, P. and Content, J. (1985b). *J. Gen. Virol.* **66**, 693–700.

Van Damme, J., De Ley, M., Van Beeumen, J., Opdenakker, G., Dayer, J. M., Billiau, A. and De Somer, P. (1985c). *Brit. J. Rheumatol.* **24**, suppl. I, 72–76.

Van Damme, J., Opdenakker, G., De Ley, M., Heremans, H. and Billiau, A. (1986). *Clin. Exp. Immunol.* **66,** 303–311.

Van Damme, J., Opdenakker, G., Cayphas, S., Van Snick, J. and Billiau, A. (1987a). *J. Exp. Med.* **165,** 914–919.

Van Damme, J., Cayphas, S., Opdenakker, G., Billiau, A. and Van Snick, J. (1987b). *Eur. J. Immunol.* **17,** 1–7.

Van Damme, J., De Ley, M., Van Snick, J., Dinarello, C. and Billiau, A. (1987c). In preparation.

Van Snick, J., Cayphas, S., Vink, A., Uyttenhove, C., Goulie, P., Rubira, M. R. and Simpson, R. J. (1986). *Proc. Natl Acad. Sci. USA.* **83,** 6979–6983.

Vilček, J., Henriksen-De Stefano, D., Siegel, D. and Le, J. (1985). *In* "The Interferon System" (F. Dianzani and G. Rossi, eds), Vol. 24, pp. 43–47. Serono Symposia.

Weissenbach, J., Chernajovsky, Y., Zeevi, M., Sandau, T. and Revel, M. (1979). *Eur. J. Biochem.* **98,** 1–8.

Weissenbach, J., Chernajovsky, Y., Zeevi, M., Shulman, L., Soreq, H., Nir, U., Wallach, D., Perricaudet, M., Tiollais, P. and Revel, M. (1980). *Proc. Natl Acad. Sci. USA* **77**, 7152–7156.

Interferon and Human Immunodeficiency Virus Infection

ROGER J. POMERANTZ AND MARTIN S. HIRSCH

Infectious Disease Unit, Massachusetts General Hospital, Boston, MA 02114, USA

The acquired immune deficiency syndrome was first described in 1981 and since then has reached epidemic proportions with cases reported on six continents (Centers for Disease Control, 1981a, b). AIDS is an immunocompromising disorder characterized by a variety of opportunistic infections and unusual tumours. Over 40,000 persons in the US alone have developed this syndrome with a 3-year mortality of over 90% (Curran, 1985). In addition, the Centers for Disease Control estimates that approximately 1.5 million individuals in the US are already infected with human immunodeficiency virus (HIV) (Curran, 1985), the aetiological agent for AIDS (Gallo *et al.*, 1984; Popovic *et al.*, 1984; Sarngadharan *et al.*, 1984). HIV (also known as LAV, HTLVIII and ARV) can also cause a variety of other disorders, ranging from an acute mononucleosis syndrome to progressive lymphadenopathy or dementia.

HIV is a retrovirus distantly related to HTLV I and II (which have been associated with the development of T cell leukaemias and lymphomas).

INTERFERON 9
ISBN 0 12 302558 3

Recent genomic studies have shown HIV to be more closely related to equine infectious anaemia, caprine arthritis-encephalitis and visna viruses (Chiu *et al.*, 1985; Gonda *et al.*, 1985; Sonigo and Alizon, 1985). These are cytopathic lentiviruses which can cause chronic disease in animals.

HIV is an encapsulated single-stranded RNA retrovirus. The first step in its replicative cycle includes binding to specific cell surface receptors. These appear to be the CD4 antigen on T cells expressing the T4 phenotype (Dalgleish *et al.*, 1984). HIV has been shown to infect monocytes as well, some of which also express CD4 antigen (Ho and Hirsch, 1986). After binding to the cell surface receptor, a process of penetration and uncoating takes place. Once in the cell, replication commences, using the viral cnzyme reverse transcriptase. Viral single-stranded RNA is used as a template with a cell-derived transfer RNA primer to synthesize complementary single-stranded DNA. Double-stranded DNA is then produced, some of which becomes integrated into the host genome as an intact provirus, using endonuclease and integrase enzymes.

The entire nucleotide sequence of integrated and unintegrated HIV proviruses has been derived (9734–9749 base pairs) (Muesing *et al.*, 1985; Ratner *et al.*, 1985; Sanchez-Pescador *et al.*, 1985; Wain-Habson *et al.*, 1985), making this the longest retrovirus genome yet sequenced. The genome is made up of a variety of genes common to retroviruses, including: *gag* (group specific antigen), *pol* (reverse transcriptase) and *env* (envelope glycoprotein). There also exist novel open-reading frames which encode for transacting factors (*tat*III and *art*) and other distinctive peptides (*sor*, 3'*orf*). Transcription of integrated HIV DNA sequences into viral messenger RNA is directed by the long terminal repeat sequences common to retroviruses. A transactivator protein, encoded by the bipartite *tat*-III gene, acts post-transcriptionally to increase levels of viral protein synthesis (Rosen *et al.*, 1986). A second transactivator protein, encoded by the gene that has been called *art* (anti-repression transactivator) or *trs*, relieves negative regulation of the messenger RNA for viral proteins (Sodroski *et al.*, 1986).

Viral proteins are produced by splicing and translation of mRNA. Many of these virus-specific proteins and glycoproteins are cleavage products of precursor polypeptides. Translation and glycosylation take place in the rough endoplasmic reticulum of the infected cell. Virus particles are assembled and released by budding through the plasma membrane in areas where viral glycoproteins congregate.

I INTERFERONS

Interferon (IFN) production *in vitro* has been shown to be depressed in a variety of immunodeficiency conditions. These include Down's syndrome, combined immunodeficiency syndrome, uraemia, and various haematological malignancies (Stiehm *et al.*, 1982). With this background, it was natural to explore the role of IFN production in AIDS. A number of studies have investigated whether circulating IFN levels could be a marker of active infection, and whether IFN-induced proteins might have a role in HIV pathogenesis. The well known antiproliferative and antiviral effects of IFNs have also led, somewhat paradoxically, to their use as antiviral and antineoplastic agents in HIV disease.

We will review the current state of knowledge regarding IFNs and HIV infection. General subtopics include: (1) IFN-α and -γ production in HIV infection and their relationship to the immunodeficient state; (2) IFN-α (acid-labile) levels in the serum of infected individuals and their use as a preclinical marker; (3) IFNs' roles as anti-HIV agents; and (4) IFN-α's role as an antineoplastic agent in Kaposi's sarcoma.

II IFN PRODUCTION AND IMMUNODEFICIENCY OF AIDS

Leukocytes from patients with AIDS characterized by opportunistic infections demonstrate deficient IFN-α production *in vitro* in response to Herpes Simplex Type I infected fibroblasts (Lopez *et al.*, 1983). Depressed IFN production was not seen in patients with only Kaposi's sarcoma and those with AIDs related complex (ARC). *In vitro* release of both IFN-α and -γ by lymphocytes from AIDS patients was similarly found to be deficient in response to CMV. This deficiency was also more marked in those patients with opportunistic infections than in those with only Kaposi's sarcoma (Epstein *et al.*, 1985). It was initially considered that this deficiency in IFN-α production might be involved in some of the various immunodeficiencies noted in AIDS. AIDS is characterized by a variety of immunological abnormalities. A prominent decrease in number and function of the T helper lymphocytes is a constant finding. Recent studies have shown that a decrease in soluble antigen recognition may be one of the major defects in the immune response (Lane *et al.*, 1985). This was found to be secondary to a lack of help rather than increased suppression. A number of other immune abnormalities have been reported in patients with AIDS, including decreased viral specific cytotoxicity, decreased natural killer activity, decreased B cell proliferation to specific antigens or mitogen (but increased spontaneous B cell proliferation and polyclonal increase in immunoglobulins), decreased production and response to interleukin 2 (IL-2) (plus decreased IL-2 receptors), decreased macrophage and monocyte functions and decreased Ia expression on macrophages (Heagy *et al.*, 1984; Bowen *et al.*, 1985).

A recent study which followed 115 patients at risk for AIDS for 45 months showed that the onset of opportunistic infection was predicted by deficiencies in both IFN-α generation *in vitro* and circulating Leu 3a+ cells. Opportunistic infections were not seen in those patients with only one of these deficiencies (Siegel *et al.*, 1986). IFN-α was found to be produced by non-T or -B large granular lymphocytes which are T lymphocyte independent. As IFN-α release is independent of the immunization state of the individual, it reflects the natural and not the adaptive component of the immune system.

It was thus relevant to test the effect of IFN-α *in vitro* in an attempt to correct some of these immune abnormalities. IFN-α reconstitution did not affect the natural killer cell activity of AIDS patients *in vitro* (Fredrick *et al.*, 1985). Natural killer cell activity, which has recently been reported to be important in HIV clearance (Ruscetti *et al.*, 1986) was, however, enhanced by IL-2 (Rook *et al.*, 1985). Virus-specific cytotoxic responses to CMV and EBV were also noted to be increased *in vitro* by IL-2 but not by IFN-β (Rook *et al.*, 1983).

IFN-γ has recently been shown to be a potent lymphokine whose production is increased by IL-2. It has been shown to increase the cytotoxic activity of macrophages (Nathan *et al.*, 1983), Ia production on macrophage surfaces (Basham and Merigan, 1983), and IL-2 receptor concentrations on T cells and macrophages (Holter *et al.*, 1986). Each of these parameters is decreased in patients with AIDS.

A variety of studies have investigated IFN-γ production in HIV infection. Initial studies showed depressed production of IFN-γ *in vitro* (Murray *et al.*, 1984), which correlated with clinical progression from ARC to AIDS (Murray *et al.*, 1985). These were performed on bulk T cell mixtures, and a recent study using isolated T8 and T4 cell preparations was unable to demonstrate a deficiency in IFN-γ production (Lane *et al.*, 1985). The reasons for these conflicting findings are not clear at the present time. One possibility is that in bulk T cell mixtures there is a suppressive subpopulation not found when the experiments were conducted with isolated T4 cell preparations. Another possibility is that there were differences in study populations. The study in which no deficiency in IFN-γ production could be found used lymphocytes from patients with only Kaposi's sarcoma and not opportunistic infections (Lane *et al.*, 1985). Therefore, these patients may have been less immunodeficient than those tested in other studies (Murray *et al.*, 1984), and may still have had intact capacity to produce IFN-γ.

Ia antigen levels are decreased on antigen presenting cells (Lane *et al.*, 1985) (macrophages and Langerhans' cells) from patients with AIDS (Heagy *et al.*, 1984; Belsito *et al.*, 1984), and IFN-γ will increase the level of Ia antigen on such cells *in vitro* (Heagy *et al.*, 1984). As the Ia antigen is important in the class II antigen T helper cell response, this deficiency in

AIDS patients may play a role in the dramatic decrease in T helper functions noted in this disease.

IFN production may also be involved in immunologically caused tissue damage in HIV infection. Visna virus, a lentivirus which causes a slow inflammatory, demyelinating disease in sheep, has been shown to infect mononuclear cells in the central nervous system. These infected macrophages secrete a soluble factor which activates T lymphocytes to produce a unique acid-stable IFN, which, in turn, increases Ia antigen expression on macrophages (Kennedy *et al.*, 1985; Narayan *et al.*, 1985). Enhanced Ia expression may lead to immunologically induced tissue damage. Thus, IFN production, either locally or systemically, may be a fundamental step in the sequence of events culminating in visna central nervous system disease (Kennedy *et al.*, 1985). Similar events may operate in the pathogenesis of HIV neurological disease (Navia *et al.*, 1986). Either IFN-γ or acid-labile IFN-α might be involved. HIV invades the central nervous system (Ho *et al.*, 1985a) and has been shown to cause a wide range of disorders. They include acute encephalitis, vacuolar myelopathy and subacute dementing encephalopathy (Navia *et al.*, 1986). The pathological lesions may be from direct viral destruction of cells, the immune response generated, or both mechanisms. Preliminary studies suggest that the amount of damage seen is disproportionate to the numbers of virus-infected cells observed. The latter cells are primarily cells of monocyte-macrophage lineage, suggesting that immunological mechanisms may be important in neuropathogenesis.

Although IFN-γ has minor effects on natural killer cell activity, it appears that IL-2 augments natural killer cell activity through an IFN-γ independent mechanism (Rook *et al.*, 1985). This has been shown both in cells from healthy individuals and in cells from AIDS patients (Rook *et al.*, 1985; Sayers *et al.*, 1986). It has recently been shown *in vitro* that natural killer activity is increased to a greater degree by IFN-α and -β than by IFN-γ (Abbud-Filho *et al.*, 1986). There also seems to be an idiosyncratic response in natural killer activity to IFN-α and -β. Different patients seem to consistently fall into high versus low responder groups (Abbud-Filho *et al.*, 1986). This makes it more complex to evaluate IFN both in *in vitro* and *in vivo* trials as an immunomodulator.

In a small recent *in vivo* study, the effect of intravenous IFN-γ on the monocytic function of patients with AIDS was evaluated. Seven patients were given intravenous IFN-γ twice weekly for 8 weeks. In 6 of 7 patients the respiratory burst of monocytes *in vitro* decreased (Pennington *et al.*, 1986). The explanation for these paradoxical results is not clear, but underscores the complexities of clinical trials of IFNs used as immunomodulators.

III IFN AS A PROGNOSTIC MARKER

Elevated IFN-α levels have been reported in sera of 17 of 17 patients with AIDS and opportunistic infections, and in 8 of 8 patients with AIDS and Kaposi's sarcoma. Elevated levels were seen in 52 of 76 healthy homosexual males and in only 1 of 24 healthy heterosexual controls (Buimovici-Klein *et al.*, 1983). The elevated levels observed in many healthy homosexual men may have been secondary to other viral illnesses (e.g. CMV, hepatitis A or B) but HIV serologies were not reported in this study.

Soon after AIDS was described, it was found that a unique IFN-α circulated in the blood of a significant percentage of these patients. It was acid-labile (inactivated by pH2) (Destefano *et al.*, 1982; Eyster *et al.*, 1983), a property characteristic of IFN-γ but not IFN-α. Although acid-labile IFN-α can be produced by normal leukocytes *in vitro,* (Balkwill *et al.,* 1983), it appears to be a minor component of IFN production in normal hosts during a viral illness (Green *et al.*, 1982). An IFN with these properties had been found previously in patients with systemic lupus erythematosis (Preble *et al.*, 1982). In one study, 65 of 138 patients with SLE had circulating acid-labile IFN-α (Preble *et al.*, 1982). In a study of patients with HIV disease, acid-labile IFN-α was found in serum of 17 of 27 patients with Kaposi's sarcoma and in 10 of 35 patients with diffuse lymphadenopathy. Only 1% of normal subjects had circulating acid-labile IFN-α (Destefano *et al.,* 1982).

In another smaller study, 3 pátients with haemophilia and AIDS were found to have this circulating acid-labile IFN-α. In two of these patients, the detection of acid-labile IFN-α preceded symptoms by many months (Eyster *et al.*, 1983).

In a third investigation, serum levels of acid-labile IFN-α were found to be elevated in 11 of 13 patients with AIDS (greater than 16 U/ml). This elevation in serum acid-labile IFN-α was not seen in 20 patients with ARC or 20 healthy homosexual men (Calabrese *et al.*, 1984). An increase in levels of serum acid-labile IFN-α antedated clinical deterioration to AIDS in 2 patients with ARC (Calabrese *et al.*, 1984).

A recent study which followed 99 initially healthy homosexual men showed that all 15 with high endogenous serum IFN-α levels developed AIDS or ARC over a 2-year follow-up. The mean time to the development of symptoms was 6.5 months. The 84 people with undetectable or very low IFN-α levels remained asymptomatic. The acid stability of the endogenous IFN-α levels in the symptomatic members of this study decreased over time. An abrupt decrease in the acid stability of the IFN-α predicted a rapid evolution to AIDS (Buimovici-Klein *et al.*, 1986). The sera from those patients with acid-labile IFN-α induced acid-labile IFN-α production from normal lymphocytes *in vitro*. It is not clear whether the acid-labile IFN in these sera produced this effect in normal lymphocytes or whether it was due to other factors in the sera (e.g. circulating immune complexes). This study suggests that high endogenous IFN-α and especially a decrease over time of its acid stability are negative prognostic indicators in HIV infection.

Another method recently used to screen for an IFN effect *in vivo* is by the measurement of 2′, 5′ oligoadenylate synthetase (Schattner *et al.*, 1981). This enzyme, induced by IFN-α, polymerizes adenosine triphosphate to yield oligoadenylic acid with 2′, 5′ phospho-diester linkages, and may be easier to detect than IFNs in peripheral blood. Local production of IFN in lymphoid tissues can increase 2′, 5′ oligoadenylate synthetase in peripheral blood mononuclear cells without increasing circulating free IFN (Preble *et al.*, 1983).

Levels of 2′, 5′ oligoadenylate synthetase were 12–14 pM per hour per 10^5 peripheral blood mononuclear cells in the 32 healthy homosexual and the 24 heterosexual controls. It averaged 129 ± 75 in 13 AIDS patients and 68 ± 84 in 33 patients with ARC. The levels of 2′, 5′ oligoadenylate synthetase were statistically different between controls and patients with AIDS ($p < 0.001$). The level was persistently elevated in 6 of 13 AIDS patients and 14 of 33 ARC patients. Four of the 14 ARC patients with elevated 2′, 5′ oligoadenylate synthetase levels subsequently developed AIDS, while none of the other 19 ARC patients developed AIDS in a 10-month follow-up period. From this preliminary study, the use of 2′, 5′ oligoadenylate synthetase as a disease marker appears promising (Read *et al.*, 1985).

This enzyme has also been used as a marker in a study of 28 AIDS patients receiving IFN-α as an antineoplastic agent in Kaposi's sarcoma (Preble *et al.*, 1985). Fifteen of 28 had high endogenous 2′, 5′ oligoadenylate synthetase levels. Exogenous IFN-α increased the level of this enzyme further in only 10 patients. This is at variance with the response seen in patients with other viral illnesses, other cancer patients, and patients with SLE (Schattner *et al.*, 1981; Preble *et al.*, 1983); these patients, although having high initial 2′, 5′ oligoadenylate synthetase levels, respond to exogenous IFN-α with a further rise in 2′, 5′ oligoadenylate synthetase levels. AIDS patients may maintain persistently elevated enzyme levels, a phenomenon also described in chronic Epstein Barr virus infection (Morag *et al.*, 1982).

Healthy homosexual controls were deficient in their ability to increase 2′, 5′ oligoadenylate synthetase levels in response to exogenous IFN-α. Studies have shown that IFN-α itself decreases IFN receptor number both *in vitro* and *in vivo* (Branea and Baglioni, 1982; Lau *et al.*, 1986). Therefore, chronically elevated IFN production in AIDS patients and possibly healthy homosexual men, secondary to HIV and/or other viral infections, may explain the diminished effect exogenous IFN-α has on inducing 2′, 5′ oligoadenylate synthetase levels.

A recent study has shown that 2′, 5′ oligoadenylate binding protein activity is 65% lower in peripheral blood lymphocytes from patients with AIDS or ARC than in those from heterosexual controls (Wu *et al.*, 1986). The 2′, 5′ oligoadenylates produced by 2′, 5′ oligoadenylate synthetase activate 2′, 5′ oligoadenylate binding protein (also known as RNase L). One would therefore have expected the 2′, 5′ oligoadenylate binding protein to be elevated in patients with AIDS, as the 2′, 5′ oligoadenylate synthetase levels are known to be high. This seeming paradox may be explained by down-regulation of 2′, 5′ oligoadenylates. The use of 2′, 5′ oligoadenylate binding protein level as an early clinical marker in HIV infection warrants further investigation.

Although we will discuss IFN and its use in Kaposi's sarcoma in more detail subsequently, it should be noted at this point that 2′, 5′ oligoadenylate synthetase levels during therapy for Kaposi's sarcoma did not predict progressive disease, whereas endogenous IFN-α levels in blood before therapy was a fair predictor of progression (Preble *et al.*, 1985). Seven of 12 patients with initially elevated IFN-α levels went on to progressive disease, as opposed to 2 of 15 with initially normal IFN-α levels (Preble *et al.*, 1985).

IV IFN AND ANTIRETROVIRAL THERAPY

In retroviral systems, IFNs have shown a variety of virus and cell-specific effects. They include effects on early events before proviral integration, post-transcriptional processing of viral precursor polypeptides (Pitha *et al.*, 1980), and viral assembly and release. *In vivo* activity has been demonstrated against both exogenous and endogenous murine leukaemia and sarcoma viruses (Pitha *et al.*, 1980; Sen *et al.*, 1984; Aboud and Hassan, 1983; Hirsch *et al.*, 1973; Gresser *et al.*, 1969). *In vitro* effects have been shown against feline and primate retroviruses (Sen *et al.*, 1984). In Moloney murine leukaemia virus systems it appears that IFN-α leads to a defect in viral assembly. An accumulation of RNA-deficient intracellular viral particles is the result (Aboud and Hassan, 1983).

Based on the above studies, certain investigators have added anti-IFN serum to an *in vitro* culture system for HIV in PBLs (Barre-Sinoussi *et al.*, 1983). There are data to suggest that anti-IFN serum used in a murine system increased retroviral production (Barre-Sinoussi *et al.*, 1983). However, no studies have been reported to demonstrate its utility in HIV cultures.

An *in vitro* study of recombinant human IFN-αA (rIFN-αA) has demonstrated a dose-related inhibitory activity against HIV replication in normal human peripheral blood mononuclear cells (Ho *et al.*, 1985b). The effects were seen at 4–64 U/ml, and there was complete inhibition of replication at

256–1024 U/ml, as measured by reverse transcriptase activity and expression of viral antigens. At these concentrations the rIFN-αA was not toxic to the target cells. It is noteworthy that 50–300 U/ml concentrations in serum can be obtained by giving 10–100 million units of rIFN-αA (Ho *et al.*, 1985b).

These results are encouraging, and clinical placebo-controlled trials comparing high dose (36×10^6 U) and low doses (3×10^6 U) of rIFN-αA given intramuscularly three times a week for 12 weeks to patients with AIDS or ARC are under way. Preliminary results in patients with Kaposi's sarcoma and AIDS suggest suppression of viremia but no change in immune parameters, measured by delayed type hypersensitivity, T cell helper to suppressor ratios, or lymphoproliferative responses (Krown *et al.*, 1986a). In a second small study, 18 patients with ARC were treated with 10×10^6 IU of rIFN-α_2 given subcutaneously three times a week for 6 months. There was no significant difference in lymph node regression or change in T helper to suppressor cell ratios in the IFN versus placebo group (Abrams *et al.*, 1986).

Further *in vitro* and *in vivo* studies in HIV infection using natural and recombinant preparations of IFN-α, -β and -γ have been performed (Table I).

TABLE I Anti-HIV Activities of Various Human IFN Preparations

IFN Preparation	PBL	T cell Lines	Monocyte Cell Lines	References
Alpha				
rIFN-αA	+	+	+	Ho *et al.* (1985); Yamamoto *et al.* (1986); Hartshorn *et al.* (in preparation)
Natural	+	+	+	Yamamoto *et al.* (1986); Hartshorn *et al.* (in preparation)
Beta				
Recombinant	+	NT	+	Hartshorn *et al.* (in preparation)
Natural	+	NT	NT	Yamamoto *et al.* (1986)
Gamma				
Recombinant	−	+/−	+	Nakashima *et al.* (1986); Yamamoto *et al.* (1986); Hartshorn *et al.* (in preparation)
Natural	−	NT	NT	Yamamoto *et al.* (1986)

NT = Not tested.

rIFN-γ leads to a dose-dependent decrease in HIV replication in HTLV-I infected T lymphocytes (MT4 cells) (Nakashima *et al.*, 1986). The effects were seen at 100–1000 U/ml, with 50–80% decrease in HIV replication as measured by immunofluorescence and cytopathic effect (Nakashima *et al.*, 1986). At these concentrations the IFN-γ did not affect the growth or viability of the target cells. The decrease in HIV replication was found to be maximum at 5 days, and HIV replication gradually increased over a longer time period. The addition of fresh IFN-γ on day 7 did not decrease viral replication further (Nakashima *et al.*, 1986).

In another study, IFN-γ showed no effect on HIV replication in peripheral blood lymphocytes, as measured by cytopathic effect and reverse transcriptase activity, at doses of 100–500 U/ml (Yamamoto *et al.*, 1986). HIV replication was decreased in a dose-dependent manner by IFN-α and -β. IFN-α decreased reverse transcriptase activity by 50% at 100 U/ml and by 77–99% at 500 U/ml. IFN-β decreased reverse transcriptase activity by 75% at 100 U/ml (Yamamoto *et al.*, 1986). Continuous replacement of IFN was necessary to maintain the antiviral effect. When only a single dose of IFN-α or -β was used, the level of viral replication after 10 days was higher in treated than in untreated cultures. This phenomenon may be explained by an IFN-induced block in viral release. Therefore, when the IFN effect waned, the preassembled virions were released at a higher concentration than in cultures never treated with IFN-α or -β (Yamamoto *et al.*, 1986). In this study, a larger dose of rIFN-α, compared to natural IFN-α preparations, was required to demonstrate an antiviral effect. As the natural IFN-α preparations are composed of a mixture of multiple subtypes of IFN-α, this suggests that it may be reasonable to evaluate combinations of multiple IFN subtypes in clinical trials (Yamamoto *et al.*, 1986).

The anti-HIV activities of other IFN preparations in a variety of cell lines have been recently investigated (Hartshorn *et al.*, in preparation). Both rIFN-αA and natural IFN-α demonstrated anti-HIV activity *in vitro* using PBLs, a T lymphocyte cell line and a monocytic cell line. rIFN-β demonstrated similar effects in PBLs and a monocyte line. IFN-γ species, both natural and recombinant, demonstrated no anti-HIV activity in PBLs. rIFN-γ showed only minimal anti-HIV activity in a T cell line, but was active against acute HIV infection of a monocyte line (U937) (Hartshorn *et al.*, in preparation).

These studies once again illustrate the complexity of IFN action as an antiviral agent. The mechanisms for the anti-HIV activities of IFNs may differ depending on the IFN preparation and/or the cell line that is used.

A further complexity has recently been added to this field by the discovery of IFN inactivator(s) in the sera of patients with AIDS (Ikossi-O'Connor *et al.*, 1986). In mixing experiments, 11 of 14 sera from patients with AIDS inactivated human leukocyte IFN-α. This was not observed with 9 control sera. This preliminary observation may have relevance in therapeutic trials of IFN preparations and in understanding the immunodeficiency of AIDS.

In vitro synergy studies with IFN-α and a variety of antiretroviral agents are promising. Synergy has been demonstrated between rIFN-αA and either phosphonoformate (Hartshorn *et al.*, 1986) or 3′ Azido-3′ deoxythymidine (AZT, BWA509U) against HIV (Hartshorn *et al.*, 1987). Both phosphonoformate and AZT are reverse transcriptase inhibitors, suggesting that agents which act at different sites of HIV replication may be useful combinations to employ (Yarchoan *et al.*, 1986; Sandstrom *et al.*, 1985; Hartshorn *et al.*, 1986). Recent controlled trials have demonstrated that AZT reduces mortality in patients with AIDS. Clinical trials of AZT in combination with IFN-α are planned. Preliminary studies also suggest synergy between rIFN-αA and ribavirin against HIV. The mechanisms of ribavirin inhibition of viral replication are not clearly defined (McCormick *et al.*, 1984). Combinations of IFN-γ and -α, which may have differing antiviral and immunomodulatory effects, also require *in vitro* and *in vivo* trials.

The lack of penetration of IFNs into the central nervous system is a drawback to their use as single antiviral agents in HIV infections. As HIV frequently invades the central nervous system and causes a variety of syndromes in the nervous system (Ho *et al.*, 1985a), the lack of penetration into the central nervous system may severely limit its use in these patients. Intrathecal administration of IFN may represent a therapeutic modality for overcoming this penetration problem.

It should be noted that the utility of IFNs alone or in combinations in HIV infection may depend on the stage of HIV infection. IFNs may find a use in less immunodeficient patients (i.e. ARC) but may be less helpful in advanced AIDS. Trials of IFNs in patients with HIV infection will therefore have to be controlled for the state of immunodeficiency of the study groups.

V IFNs AND KAPOSI'S SARCOMA

IFN have been shown to have a variety of antiproliferative effects. They have been found to induce regression in a variety of tumours, including breast carcinoma, multiple myeloma, lymphoma, osteosarcoma and hairy cell leukaemia (Stiehm *et al.*, 1982). With the recent production of recombinant human IFNs, large sources of pure species of IFN have become available for trials. The use of IFN-α in patients with Kaposi's sarcoma and AIDS was a logical therapeutic trial. The antiviral effects of IFN-α may be useful in this disease, because of the possible viral aetiology of Kaposi's sarcoma (Boldogh *et al.*, 1981).

A number of clinical trials have been performed with both natural and recombinant IFN-α preparations in Kaposi's sarcoma. Patient populations have differed in severity of disease, and therapeutic results have varied. In one study 30 patients with Kaposi's sarcoma were treated with lymphoblastoid IFN-α given intramuscularly daily for 28 days at doses of 7.5, 15 and 28 MU/m^2 (Gelmann *et al.*, 1985). Because of side-effects, which included reversible granulocytopenia, headache, fever, chills, myalgias and peripheral neuropathy, the higher dose was later dropped from the protocol. Three patients had partial and 4 had minor responses to the therapy. This is at variance with the 30 and 42% partial or complete response rate in two older studies in which rIFN-αA was used. This poor response rate in the later study may be because of a difference in efficacy between natural and recombinant IFN-α or, more likely, because the T4/T8 ratios were higher in patients in the older studies (Krown *et al.*, 1983; Groopman *et al.*, 1984). This higher average T4/T8 ratio is an indicator of a less immunodeficient patient population, and one therefore more likely to respond positively to therapy. The use of a relatively high T helper to suppressor cell ratio as a positive prognostic indicator has been shown in a group of patients with AIDS and Kaposi's sarcoma (Taylor *et al.*, 1986). In the recent study, prognostic indicators of progressive disease included low total lymphocyte counts, prior opportunistic infections and endogenous levels of acid-labile IFN-α prior to treatment. The poor prognosis in patients with endogenous acid-labile IFN may be secondary to decreased natural killer activity or down-regulation of IFN receptors.

A recent study of 19 patients with AIDS and Kaposi's sarcoma showed only 2 patients obtaining tumour regression when treated with lymphoblastoid IFN (Fredrick *et al.*, 1985). No effects on active CMV or EBV infections were noted at either the high (15×10^6 U/m^2 IM $\times$ 20 days) or low (7.5×10^6 U/m^2 IM) doses. It should be noted that natural killer activity decreased in 11 of 14 patients during treatment. This decrease in natural killer activity has been seen in other disease states treated with prolonged IFN therapy (Maluish *et al.*, 1983; Kelly *et al.*, 1984).

A recently completed study evaluated the use of rIFN-α_{2a} in patients with Kaposi's sarcoma and AIDS. Thirty-eight per cent of 78 patients had partial or complete response. The regiment was 36–54 $\times$ 10^6 U IM daily for 4 weeks followed by three times a week for 4 additional weeks. A low-dose regimen (3×10^6 U IM daily) was not effective. Responders to therapy had fewer opportunistic infections and better pretreatment immune status than nonresponders. The immune status of the responders did not improve during therapy. The responders to therapy also differed from the nonresponders in the lack of endogenous pretreatment serum IFN activity (Krown *et al.*, 1986b).

IFN-α remains an important investigational agent against Kaposi's sarcoma in AIDS patients. Controlled clinical trials of IFN-α and combination trials of IFN-α and other chemotherapeutic agents are under way. The chemotherapeutic agents with the most promise include Vincristine, Vinblastine, Etoposide (VP16) and Daunorubicin.

VI CONCLUSIONS

A number of abnormalities in the IFN system have been described in patients with AIDS, ARC or asymptomatic HIV infection. Production of IFN-α and -γ by leukocytes in response to antigens may be reduced, with secondary effects on macrophage and lymphocyte function. An acid-labile IFN-α is detected in the circulation of many HIV-infected individuals, and may play a role in immunopathogenesis by down-regulating IFN receptors, decreasing natural killer cells, or increasing Ia antigen expression. Moreover, detection of acid-labile IFN-α or its induced enzyme, 2′, 5′ oligoadenylate synthetase, in the circulation appears to be useful as a clinical marker of poor prognosis. The utility of these measurements when compared to other assays, e.g. enumeration of T helper lymphocytes or T cell subsets, remains unclear.

IFN-α has anti-HIV activity *in vitro*, and is under study in a number of clinical trials among patients infected with this virus. The lack of central nervous system penetration of IFNs is a drawback to their use as single antiviral agents in HIV infections, which usually involve the brain and spinal cord. Intrathecal administration of IFNs, or combination with other antiviral agents, may ameliorate this problem. Synergism of IFN-α with certain reverse transcriptase inhibitors, including azidothymidine, has been demonstrated *in vitro*.

Trials of various IFN-α preparations in patients with AIDS-related Kaposi's sarcoma have shown antitumour activity in 10–42%. Response appears to be related to the integrity of the immune response at the time of therapy. Detectable levels of circulating acid-labile IFN-α are a poor prognostic sign for response of Kaposi's sarcoma to exogenous IFNs.

The clinical response of HIV-infected patients to IFNs, alone or in combination, may depend on many factors, including the severity of immunological impairment, the degree of neurological involvement, the viral burden, and many as yet unrecognized factors, including individual variation. We have only begun to explore the complexities of interactions between HIV and the IFN system, and further surprises undoubtedly lie ahead.

REFERENCES

Abbud-Filho, M., Ransil, B. and Kelley, B. (1986). *Clin. Imm. Immunopath.* **39**, 264.
Aboud, M. and Hassan, Y. (1983). *J. Virol.* **45**, 489–495.

Abrams, D., Andes, W., Kisner, D. *et al.* (1986). "A trial of alpha 2 interferon in a benign reactive lymphadenopathic syndrome." International Conference on AIDS, June 23, 1986, Paris (abstract).

Balkwill, F., Griffin, D., Band, H. and Beverly, P. (1983). *J. Exp. Med.* **157**, 1059.

Barre-Sinoussi, F., Chermann, J., Rey, F. *et al.* (1983). *Science* **220**, 868.

Basham, T. and Merigan, T. (1983). *J. Immunol.* **130**, 1492.

Belsito, D., Sanchez, M., Baer, R. *et al.* (1984). *N. Eng. J. Med.* **310**, 1279.

Boldogh, I., Beth, E., Huang, E. *et al.* (1981). *Int. J. Cancer* **28**, 469.

Bowen, D., Lane, H. and Fauci, A. (1985). *Ann. Int. Med.* **103**, 704.

Branea, A. and Baglioni, C. (1982). *J. Biol. Chem.* **257**, 13197.

Buimovici-Klein, E., Lange, M. and Klein, R. (1983). *Lancet* **ii**, 344 (Letter).

Buimovici-Klein, E., Lange, M., Klein, R. *et al.* (1986). *AIDS Research* **2**, 99.

Calabrese, L., Profitt, M., Gupta, M. *et al.* (1984). *AIDS Research* **1**, 423.

Centers for Disease Control. (1981a). *Morbid. Mortal. Weekly Rep.* **30,** 250–252.

Centers for Disease Control. (1981b). *Morbid. Mortal. Weekly Rep.* **30**, 305–307.

Chiu, I., Yaniv, A., Dahlberg, J. *et al.* (1985). *Nature* **317**, 366–368.

Curran, J. W. (1985). "The Epidemiology and Prevention of AIDS." International Conference on Acquired Immunodeficiency Syndrome, Atlanta, April 1, pp. 14–17.

Dalgleish, A., Beverly, P., Clapham, P. *et al.* (1984). *Nature* **312**, 763–766.

Destefano, E., Friedman, R., Friedman-Kien, A. *et al.* (1982). *J. Infect. Dis.* **146**, 451.

Epstein, J., Fredrick, W., Rook, A. *et al.* (1985). *J. Infect. Dis* **152**, 727.

Eyster, N., Goedert, J., Poon, M. and Preeble, D. (1983). *N. Engl. J. Med.* **309**, 583.

Fredrick, W., Epstein, J., Gelmann, E. *et al.* (1985). *J. Infect. Dis.* **152**, 112.

Fredrick, W., Epstein, J. and Gelmann, E. (1985). *J. Infect. Dis.* **152**, 162.

Gallo, R. C., Salahuddin, S. Z., Popovic, M. *et al.* (1984). *Science* **224,** 500–503.

Gelmann, E., Preble, D., Steis, R. *et al.* (1985). *Am. J. Med.* **78**, 737.

Gonda, M. A., Wong-Staal, F., Gallo, R. C. *et al.* (1985). *Science* **227**, 173–177.

Green, J., Charette, R., Yeh, T.-J. and Smith, C. (1982). *J. Infect Dis.* **145**, 837.

Gresser, I., Coppey, J. and Bovrali, C. (1969). *J. Natl Cancer Inst.* **43**, 1083.

Groopman, J., Gottlieb, M., Goodman, J. *et al.* (1984). *Ann. Int. Med.* **100**, 671.

Hartshorn, K., Sandstrom, E., Neumeyer, D. *et al.* (1986). *Antimicrob. Ag. Chem.* **30**, 189.

Hartshorn, K., Vogt, M., Chou, T. C. *et al.* (1987) *Antimicrob. Ag. Chem.* **31,** 168.

Hartshorn, K. and Hirsch, M. *et al.* (1987). Manuscript in preparation.

Heagy, W., Kelley, V., Strom, T. *et al.* (1984). *J. Clin. Invest.* **74**, 2089.

Hirsch, M., Ellis, D., Proffit, M. and Black, P. (1973). *Nature New Biology* **244**, 102.

Ho, D., Rota, T. and Hirsch, M. (1986). *J. Clin. Invest.* **97**, 1.

Ho, D., Rota, T., Schooley, R. *et al.* (1985a) *N. Engl. J. Med.* **313**, 1493.

Ho, D. D., Rota, T., Kaplan, J. *et al.* (1985b). *Lancet* **i**, 602–604.

Holter, W., Grunow, R., Stockinger, H. and Knapp, W. (1986). *J. Immunol.* **136**, 2176.

Ikossi-O'Connor, M., Chadha, K., Lillie, M. *et al.* (1986). *Am. J. Med.* **81**, 783.

Kelly, A., Schooley, R., Rubin, R. and Hirsch, M. (1984). *Clin. Immun. Immunopath.* **32**, 20.

Kennedy, P., Narayan, O., Ghotbi, Z. *et al.* (1985). *J. Exp. Med.* **162**, 1970.

Krown, S., Real, F., Cunningham-Rundles, S. *et al.* (1983). *N. Engl. J. Med.* **308**, 1071.

Krown, S., Real, F., Gold, S. *et al.* (1986a). "Therapeutic trials of interferon alpha-2a in AIDS related Kaposi's sarcoma." International Conference on AIDS, June 23, 1986, Paris (abstract).

Krown, S., Real, F., Vadhan-Raj, S. *et al.* (1986b). *Cancer* **57**, 1662.
Lane, H. C., Depper, J., Green, W. *et al.* (1985). *N. Engl. J. Med.* **313**, 79.
Lau, A., Hannigan, G., Freedman, M. and Williams, B. (1986). *J. Clin. Invest.* **77**, 1632.
Lopez, C., Fitzgerald, P. and Siegel, F. (1983). *JID* **148**, 962.
Maluish, A., Ortaldo, J., Conlon, J. *et al.* (1983). *J. Immunol.* **131**, 503.
McCormick, J., Mitchell, S., Getchell, J. *et al.* (1984). *Lancet* **i**, 1367–1369.
Morag, A., Tobi, M., Ravid, Z. *et al.* (1982). *Lancet* **i**, 744 (Letter).
Muesing, M. A., Smith, D. M., Cabradilla, C. D. *et al.* (1985). *Nature* **313**, 450–458.
Murray, H., Rubin, B., Masur, H. and Roberts, R. (1984). *N. Eng. J. Med.* **310**, 883.
Murray, H., Hillman, J., Rubin, B. *et al.* (1985). *N. Engl. J. Med.* **313**, 1504.
Nakashima, H., Yoshida, T., Harada, S. and Yamamoto, N. (1986). *Int. J. Cancer* **38**, 433.
Nathan, C., Murray, H., Wiebe, M. and Rubin, B. (1983). *J. Exp. Med.* **158**, 670.
Narayan, D., Shefter, D., Clements, J. and Tennekoon, G. (1985). *J. Exp. Med.* **112**, 1954.
Navia, B., Eun-Sook, C., Petito, C. and Price, R. (1986). *Ann. Neurol.* **19**, 525.
Pennington, J., Groopman, J., Small, G. *et al.* (1986). *J. Infect. Dis.* **153**, 609.
Pitha, P., Fernie, B., Maldarelli, T. *et al.* (1980). *J. Gen. Virol.* **46**, 97.
Popovic, M., Sarngadharan, M. G., Read, E. and Gallo, R. C. (1984). *Science* **224**, 497–500.
Preble, D., Black, R., Friedman, R. *et al.* (1982). *Science* **216**, 429.
Preble, O., Rothko, K., Kippel, J. *et al.* (1983). *J. Exp. Med.* **157**, 2140.
Preble, O., Rook, A., Steis, R. *et al.* (1985). *J. Infect. Dis.* **152**, 457.
Ratner, L., Hazeltine, W., Patrarca, R. *et al.* (1985). *Nature* **313**, 277–284.
Read, S., Williams, B., Contes, R. *et al.* (1985). *J. Infect. Dis.* **152**, 466.
Rook, A., Masur, H., Lane, H. *et al.* (1983). *J. Clin. Invest.* **72**, 398.
Rook, A., Hooks, J., Quinnan, G. *et al.* (1985). *J. Immunol.* **134**, 1503.
Rosen, C., Sodroski, J., Goh, W. C. *et al.* (1986). *Nature* **319**, 555.
Ruscetti, F., Mikovits, J., Kalyanaraman, V. *et al.* (1986). *J. Immunol.* **136**, 3619.
Sanchez-Pescador, R., Power, M. D., Ball, P. J. *et al.* (1985). *Science* **227**, 484–492.
Sandstrom, E., Byington, R., Kaplan, J. and Hirsch, M. S. (1985). *Lancet* **i**, 1480–1482.
Sarngadharan, M. G., Popovic, M., Bruch, L. *et al.* (1984). *Science* **224**, 506–508.
Sayers, T., Mason, A. and Ortaldo, J. (1986). *J. Immunol.* **136**, 2176.
Schattner, A., Wallach, D., Merlin, G. *et al.* (1981). *Lancet* **2**, 497.
Sen, G. C., Herz, R., Davatelis, V. and Pestka, S. (1984). *J. Virol.* **50**, 445.
Siegel, F., Lopez, C., Fitzgerald, P. *et al.* (1986). *J. Clin. Invest.* **78**, 115.
Sodroski, J., Goh, W. C., Rosen, C. *et al.* (1986). *Nature* **321**, 412.
Sonigo, P. and Alizon, M. (1985). *Cell* **42**, 369–382.
Stiehm, E., Kronenberg, L., Rosenblatt, H. *et al.* (1982). *Ann. Int. Med.* **96**, 80.
Taylor, J., Afrasiabi, R., Fahey, J. *et al.* (1986). *Blood* **67**, 666.
Wain-Habson, S., Sonigo, P., Danos, D. *et al.* (1985). *Cell* **48**, 9–17.
Wu, J., Chiao, J. and Maayen, S. (1986). *AIDS Research* **2**, 127.
Yamamoto, J., Barre-Sinoussi, F., Bolton, V. *et al.* (1986). *J. Interferon Research* **6**, 143.
Yarchoan, R., Weinhold, K., Lyerly, H. *et al.* (1986). *Lancet* **i**, 575–580.